DISEASES AND DISORDERS

MIGRAINES
MANAGING SEVERE HEADACHES

By Jennifer Lombardo

Portions of this book originally appeared in *Migraines* by Anne K. Brown.

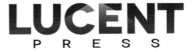

Published in 2019 by
Lucent Press, an Imprint of Greenhaven Publishing, LLC
353 3rd Avenue
Suite 255
New York, NY 10010

Designer: Deanna Paternostro
Editor: Jennifer Lombardo

Cataloging-in-Publication Data

Names: Lombardo, Jennifer.
Title: Migraines: managing severe headaches / Jennifer Lombardo.
Description: New York : Lucent Press, 2019. | Series: Diseases and disorders | Includes glossary and index.
Identifiers: ISBN 9781534563612 (pbk.) | ISBN 9781534563599 (library bound) | ISBN 9781534563605 (ebook)
Subjects: LCSH: Migraine–Juvenile literature.
Classification: LCC RC392.L63 2019 | DDC 616.8'4912–dc23

Printed in the United States of America

CPSIA compliance information: Batch #BS18KL: For further information contact Greenhaven Publishing LLC, New York, New York at 1-844-317-7404.

Please visit our website, www.greenhavenpublishing.com. For a free color catalog of all our high-quality books, call toll free 1-844-317-7404 or fax 1-844-317-7405.

CONTENTS

FOREWORD   **4**

INTRODUCTION
More Than Just a Headache   **6**

CHAPTER ONE
Understanding Migraines   **8**

CHAPTER TWO
Differences Among Migraines   **28**

CHAPTER THREE
Managing Migraines   **44**

CHAPTER FOUR
Treating Migraines   **58**

CHAPTER FIVE
Continuing Research   **80**

NOTES   **90**
GLOSSARY   **94**
ORGANIZATIONS TO CONTACT   **95**
FOR MORE INFORMATION   **97**
INDEX   **99**
PICTURE CREDITS   **103**
ABOUT THE AUTHOR   **104**

FOREWORD

Illness is an unfortunate part of life, and it is one that is often misunderstood. Thanks to advances in science and technology, people have been aware for many years that diseases such as the flu, pneumonia, and chicken pox are caused by viruses and bacteria. These diseases all cause physical symptoms that people can see and understand, and many people have dealt with these diseases themselves. However, sometimes diseases that were previously unknown in most of the world turn into epidemics and spread across the globe. Without an awareness of the method by which these diseases are spread—through the air, through human waste or fluids, through sexual contact, or by some other method—people cannot take the proper precautions to prevent further contamination. Panic often accompanies epidemics as a result of this lack of knowledge.

Knowledge is power in the case of mental disorders, as well. Mental disorders are just as common as physical disorders, but due to a lack of awareness among the general public, they are often stigmatized. Scientists have studied them for years and have found that they are generally caused by hormonal imbalances in the brain, but they have not yet determined with certainty what causes those imbalances or how to fix them. Because even mild mental illness is stigmatized in Western society, many people prefer not to talk about it.

Chronic pain disorders are also not well understood—even by researchers—and do not yet have foolproof treatments. People who have a mental disorder or a disease or disorder that causes them to feel chronic pain can be the target of uninformed opinions. People who do not have these disorders sometimes struggle to understand how difficult it can be to deal with the symptoms. These disorders are often termed "invisible illnesses" because no one can see the symptoms; this leads many people to doubt that they exist or are serious problems. Additionally, people who have an undiagnosed disorder may understand that they are experiencing the world in a different way than their peers, but they have no one to turn to for answers.

Misinformation about all kinds of ailments is often spread through personal anecdotes, social media, and even news sources. This series aims to present accurate information about both physical and mental conditions so young adults will have a better understanding of them. Each volume discusses the symptoms of a particular disease or disorder, ways it is currently being treated, and the research that is being done to understand it further. Advice for people who may be suffering from a disorder is included, as well as information for their loved ones about how best to support them.

With fully cited quotes, a list of recommended books and websites for further research, and informational charts, this series provides young adults with a factual introduction to common illnesses. By learning more about these ailments, they will be better able to prevent the spread of contagious diseases, show compassion to people who are dealing with invisible illnesses, and take charge of their own health.

MORE THAN JUST A HEADACHE

Nearly everyone in the world has had a headache at one point, and most are easy to deal with. Some are so mild that people can continue their daily activities even while they have one. Some go away on their own, while others can easily be treated with over-the-counter (OTC) pain medications such as ibuprofen (Advil) and acetaminophen (Tylenol). However, migraines are not like typical headaches. They are much more painful, last longer, often come with side effects such as nausea and vision changes, and generally require rest and prescription medication as treatment. For some people, even medications do not work, and they must simply wait until the migraine passes on its own.

Approximately 37 million Americans suffer from migraines. Most people cannot function normally when they have a migraine, which sometimes causes them to miss work or social events. Severe migraines can send a patient to bed for two to three days at a time. Many of those sufferers experience several migraines each year, and some have more than one per month. Not every migraine is exactly the same, but individuals' migraines tend to follow the same pattern repeatedly. For example, if someone's migraines include vision changes, they are likely to have this symptom almost every time they get a migraine.

These intense headaches have gained greater public discussion in recent years. Migraines have become recognized and accepted as a real medical condition

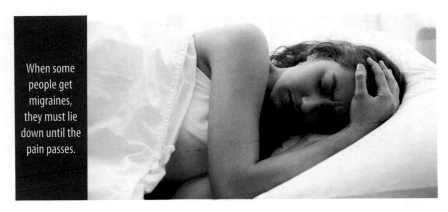

When some people get migraines, they must lie down until the pain passes.

and not simply as an overreaction on the part of a patient. As more people have come to understand their own migraines, they have openly revealed their personal experiences, sometimes as a means to help others. A number of celebrities suffer or have suffered from migraines, including tennis star Serena Williams, actor Ben Affleck, and football Hall of Famer Terrell Davis, who was forced to miss the second quarter of Super Bowl XXXII due to a sudden migraine. Artist Vincent van Gogh, author Lewis Carroll, and scientist Charles Darwin were also victims of migraines. Migraines do not discriminate in their attacks and may affect anyone at any time.

Migraines are being studied extensively in the medical community. Researchers do not completely understand what happens in the brain during a migraine, and they have yet to find a way to permanently prevent them.

Nonetheless, new research and new medical technology offer hope to migraine sufferers. With advances in technology that let researchers analyze the brain, doctors are getting closer to understanding the process of a migraine. When the mechanism that starts a migraine is eventually discovered, people prone to migraines might look forward to a cure for their headaches or a method of prediction or prevention that could forever change their lives for the better.

CHAPTER ONE

UNDERSTANDING MIGRAINES

Migraines have been misunderstood for a long time, even by some medical professionals. People who have never experienced one sometimes have trouble imagining how painful they are, so a person who gets migraines may encounter people who wrongly believe they are either exaggerating their pain or too sensitive to what others see as a bearable amount of pain. This is frustrating for them, especially when it comes from doctors who do not take them seriously. Fortunately, as migraines have become the focus of more studies, doctors have gained a better idea of how to diagnose and treat them and are less likely to dismiss their patients than they might have been in the past.

Not all headaches are migraines. Some people substitute the word "migraine" for any type of headache, especially one that is more painful than they ordinarily experience. This can lead to confusion and misunderstanding of true migraines. Doctors and researchers have come to understand that migraines have a set of very specific symptoms and often occur under specific circumstances. Anyone who has ever had a migraine can agree that a migraine is far different from an ordinary headache.

Labeling Different Kinds of Headaches

Because headaches are so common and come in so many different types, doctors divide them into two distinct categories: secondary headaches and primary headaches. This helps doctors understand the cause of a headache and how to treat it.

Understanding the different types of headaches becomes a little easier by being able to distinguish

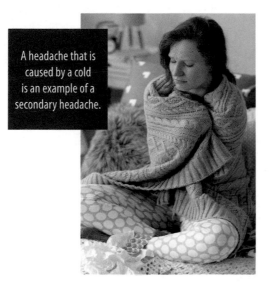

A headache that is caused by a cold is an example of a secondary headache.

between a symptom and a disease. A symptom is a physical ailment that appears because of an illness; for example, sneezing, coughing, headache, and a stuffy nose are symptoms of a cold. Bright red, itchy bumps are a symptom of chicken pox. A disease, on the other hand, is the root cause of an illness. Mumps, influenza, and measles are diseases that cause a variety of different symptoms in patients. Headaches can be symptoms, but they can also be a disease. This distinction is extremely important to a doctor's diagnosis, and it is the distinction that separates secondary headaches from primary headaches.

Headaches That Are Symptoms

Doctors describe a secondary headache as any headache that is the symptom of another disease. Secondary headaches are triggered by an illness or injury. Migraines do not fall into this group because they are not caused by diseases or other conditions.

Doctors sometimes use headaches to diagnose a disease. They must make certain to treat the disease, not just the headache. If a patient complains of recurring headaches, for example, a doctor would be unwise to continually suggest aspirin and bed rest. By asking

Asking the Right Questions

Doctors ask many questions when trying to diagnose a headache. Below is a list of common questions:

- When was your first headache? How long do the headaches last? How often do the headaches occur?
- Where is the pain felt? What type of pain is felt?
- What makes the headache better, and what makes it worse?
- Do medications help?
- Have you ever had a blow to the head?
- What surgeries or illnesses have you had?
- How old were you when the headaches began?
- What other symptoms accompany the headaches?
- What triggers the headaches?
- Do any family members suffer from headaches?

questions about the headache and other symptoms, a doctor might determine that a patient has a condition as mild as a head cold or as serious as a brain tumor. For secondary headaches, treating the headache will not cure the disease, but treating the disease will almost certainly cure the headache. However, doctors may treat the headache at the same time as the disease to help relieve the pain temporarily; for instance, if the headache is caused by a sinus infection, the doctor may tell the patient they can take aspirin to make their head feel better while they are waiting for their antibiotics to get rid of their infection.

Secondary headaches can accompany a wide range of illnesses. The symptoms of these diseases help distinguish these headaches from migraines. Secondary headaches might be symptoms of the following diseases and injuries:

- rheumatoid arthritis, which causes swelling

and pain in the joints, such as fingers, knees, and elbows
- meningitis, an infection in the fluid that surrounds the brain, which is generally signaled by a severe headache and a high fever
- brain tumor or other brain abnormality
- hemorrhage, or bleeding inside the brain
- concussion or blow to the head, such as from a sports injury or accident
- many other ailments, such as a cold, flu, allergies, and sinus infection

In addition, people who are addicted to illegal drugs, alcohol, or caffeine may experience headaches when they try to quit using these substances.

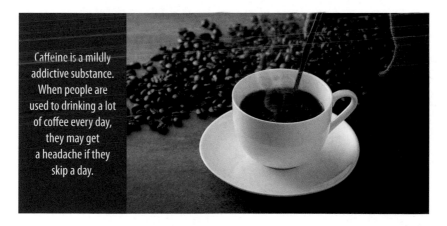

Caffeine is a mildly addictive substance. When people are used to drinking a lot of coffee every day, they may get a headache if they skip a day.

Doctors can often determine the cause of secondary headaches by understanding other symptoms or situations in the patient's life. By comparing these with the symptoms of a migraine, doctors can also quickly recognize that these types of headaches are not migraines.

When Headaches Are the Main Problem

The other category of headaches—primary headaches—includes migraines. Primary headaches are not related to other diseases or medical problems.

A primary headache is recognized as the ailment that needs treatment. Rather than treating an underlying disease and thus curing a headache, doctors attempt to cure primary headaches by understanding and targeting the headache directly.

Primary headaches are unpleasant, but they cause no damage to the rest of the body. While secondary headaches might accompany an ailment or disease that could be fatal to the patient, such as a brain tumor, aneurysm, or stroke, primary headaches are not generally life threatening. Doctors and researchers recognize four types of primary headaches: tension headaches, cluster headaches, new daily persistent headaches (NDPH), and migraines.

People who are under stress are likely to get a tension headache, which is also sometimes called a tension-type headache. According to the Cleveland Clinic, anywhere from 30 to 80 percent of the American population gets occasional tension headaches, but only 3 percent have chronic tension headaches, which means they occur more than 15 days every month. These headaches generally cause dull, aching pain in the forehead or along the sides and back of the head, along with a feeling of pressure. The pain sometimes flows down the neck and shoulders. Such a headache might last a few hours or might continue for several days. One of the reasons why migraines and tension headaches are confused is the length of the headache; both can last for several days. Lack of sleep, poor nutrition, skipping meals, poor posture, lack of physical activity, and anxiety can all contribute to tension headaches, but the exact cause is still unknown. Some researchers believe it is due to increased pain sensitivity, but more research must be done to prove or disprove this theory. The tension headache gets its name from the muscle tension that often accompanies this headache. Muscle tension in the face, jaw, neck, and shoulders is not the cause of a tension headache, as was once thought, but is another symptom of the underlying stress that can cause this headache.

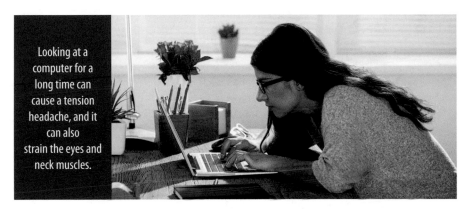

Looking at a computer for a long time can cause a tension headache, and it can also strain the eyes and neck muscles.

The Mayo Clinic described the differences between a tension headache and a migraine:

> *Unlike some forms of migraine, tension headaches usually aren't associated with visual disturbances, nausea or vomiting. Although physical activity typically aggravates migraine pain, it doesn't make tension headache pain worse. An increased sensitivity to either light or sound can occur with a tension headache, but these aren't common symptoms.*[1]

Another type of primary headache is the cluster headache. Cluster headaches bring on a strong pain around one eye or one side of the head. People who have experienced them generally say the pain is the worst they have ever felt. They get their name from their pattern: They occur in clusters, or small groups. A person will be pain-free for a while—anywhere from several weeks to a year, depending on the person—and then develop a headache at about the same time every day. Some people experience several in a day. Each headache generally lasts between 15 minutes and 3 hours, and each cluster period generally lasts for about 6 to 12 weeks. The cluster pattern helps distinguish these headaches from migraines, although cluster headaches may share some of the same symptoms, such as sensitivity to light and sound. Like other primary headaches, the exact cause of cluster headaches is uncertain, but experts suggest it is related to the body's internal clock, since most cluster headaches occur at night. Unlike tension headaches and migraines, they are generally not triggered by outside factors such as stress or a particular food, although alcohol may make them worse.

NDPH is a headache syndrome in which headaches start seemingly at random and persist for three months or more. Although the pain may get stronger or weaker, it is there every day. These headaches feel similar to tension or migraine headaches. Doctors are unsure what causes them.

Migraine headaches have a unique set of symptoms. A migraine is a headache that lasts from 4 to 72 hours if it is left untreated and is severe enough to prevent the patient from taking part in normal activities. A migraine gives a pulsing sensation and generally causes pain on only one side of the head. A common characteristic of migraines is sensitivity to light and sound—bright lights or loud noises might be painful, and a patient might seek out a quiet, dark room. Migraines are known to cause auras in some patients—strange flashes of light or other visual disturbances, such as blind spots—but most people do not experience auras when they get a migraine. Another common characteristic is nausea or vomiting.

Understanding Migraine Symptoms

Migraines have four distinct phases, although not everyone experiences all four. Additionally, a person may experience different types of migraines, which sometimes makes it difficult for them to explain their symptoms to a doctor.

The first stage is the prodrome—warning signs that occur one or two days before the actual migraine. They are vague symptoms that are easily mistaken for something else. A patient may brush aside these symptoms and blame them on stress, lack of sleep, a virus, or overwork. A person who has had many migraines, however, might know what to expect during this phase and may correctly predict that a migraine is beginning. This may help them plan ahead and avoid scheduling activities they may have to cancel later. Symptoms of the prodrome may include:

- *Constipation*
- *Mood changes, from depression to euphoria*
- *Food cravings*
- *Neck stiffness*
- *Increased thirst and urination*
- *Frequent yawning*[2]

Again, not everyone experiences a prodrome; sometimes migraines come on without warning.

The second stage is the aura. Auras are a complicated topic, and they are frequently misunderstood. Only about one-quarter of migraines come with an aura; it is more common not to experience one. The most common aura symptoms are visual disturbances such as flashes of light, sparkling dots, or bright, wavy lines that interfere with a person's vision, similar to the afterimage of a camera flash. Auras may cause blurry vision or flashes of light. Sometimes the aura begins as a bright, shimmering speck that grows larger and larger. People who experience auras report that they generally begin 20 to 60 minutes before the start of the migraine, but they may appear as early as two days before a headache. The auras typically last about 10 to 25 minutes, but they can last as long as 60 minutes.

Deborah Weaver has had numerous migraines, and

her auras lead to temporary blindness, known as sco-
toma. Weaver explained,

> *It starts with a flash of light, then I get a tiny blur-*
> *ry spot in the middle of my vision. Then I lose my*
> *vision around the outside edges, and the blindness*
> *narrows down until I can see only a small spot. I*
> *lose [that small spot of vision] and I can't see any-*
> *thing for 20 to 40 minutes. I can't drive, read, or*
> *walk across a room. I can make out shapes and col-*
> *ors, so I'm not completely blind, but I can't focus on*
> *anything. After my vision comes back, my eyes are*
> *sore but I can function again.*[3]

Some auras also include sensory symptoms. In the
past, many doctors called these complex migraines,
but this term is no longer preferred; instead, they
are simply included in the category of migraine with
aura. When these symptoms occur, they are often
similar to the symptoms of a stroke or transient ischemic attack (TIA)—previously called a mini-stroke,
although medical experts no longer prefer this term.
A stroke is a life-threatening condition caused by an
interruption of blood flow to the brain; a TIA is a
temporary blockage of a blood vessel in the brain that
does not damage the brain but is a strong warning
sign of a future stroke. Although migraines with aura
are not deadly, they can be scary to people who do not
know what is going on. The symptoms may include
muscle weakness, speech problems such as word slur-
ring or difficulty saying the correct word, inability to
concentrate, numbness or a feeling of pins and needles on one side of the face and body, and auditory
hallucinations—hearing things no one else can hear.
Sometimes this kind of migraine occurs without pain.

The difference between a migraine with aura and a
stroke or TIA is that, while all three are the result of
changes in blood flow in the brain, the changes occur
differently in a migraine than in a stroke or TIA. A

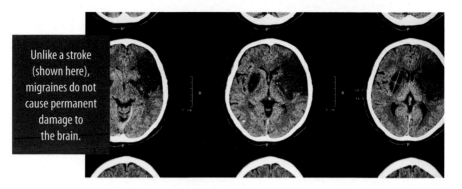

Unlike a stroke (shown here), migraines do not cause permanent damage to the brain.

migraine does not damage the brain the way a stroke does and is not an indicator of a future stroke the way a TIA is. However, people who experience these symptoms for the first time should get to a hospital immediately, as it is difficult to tell without medical tests what the source of the problem is.

The third stage of a migraine is the attack. This is when a person experiences the intense pain, sensitivity to light (photophobia) and sound (phonophobia), nausea and vomiting, dizziness, and blurred vision that make it difficult to participate in normal activities. Most people take their medication and lie down in a dark room until the attack passes. The headache might occur in a number of different forms. Most often, the pain is described as pounding or throbbing. In most attacks, the headache is limited to one side of the head, but in some cases, headache pain is on both sides of the head. The pain is often concentrated on the forehead. The headache almost always becomes worse when the patient bends over or takes part in physical activity—even mild activity such as walking to the bathroom.

A variety of minor symptoms might accompany migraines; these symptoms vary widely from person to person. Although some people will not experience any such symptoms, others might endure several at once. These symptoms include sweating, chills, pale skin, diarrhea, bloating, constipation, a stiff neck, lack of concentration, anxiety, lightheadedness, and irritability. This wide range of symptoms can even differ from one headache to the next in the same person, and this fact sometimes adds to the difficulty in diagnosing a migraine.

The fourth stage is the postdrome. This happens after the attack passes; many people feel exhausted, although some feel refreshed or energized. Other symptoms may include confusion, moodiness, weakness, and continued sensitivity to light and sound.

Examining the Brain

Because headaches affect different parts of the head and vary in severity, a reasonable assumption is that different headaches are caused by different structures inside the head. Researchers have concluded that this is true—the various primary headaches are triggered in different parts of the brain. For migraines, these include the cerebrum, cerebellum, brain stem, meninges, and thalamus.

Each part of the brain is responsible for controlling different aspects of human behavior. The cerebrum,

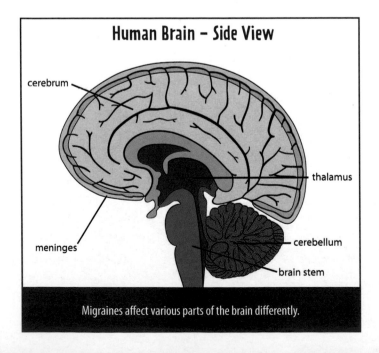

Human Brain – Side View

cerebrum

thalamus

meninges

cerebellum

brain stem

Migraines affect various parts of the brain differently.

or cerebral cortex, is the largest part of the brain, and it contains nerve centers associated with sensory and motor functions. When someone hears a bird chirping, tastes chocolate, writes a message, or kicks a ball, the cerebrum is at work. The cerebrum is also responsible for higher mental functions, such as memory and reasoning. If someone memorizes a telephone number or solves a riddle, the cerebrum is doing its job.

The cerebellum is a smaller part of the brain at the back of the head, and it is home to nerve centers that regulate balance and coordinate voluntary movement. The cerebellum reacts to sensory information and is able to control muscles attached to the skeleton. This allows arms, legs, fingers, and toes to work together and produce coordinated movement. When someone pulls a hand away from a hot stove, the cerebellum is controlling the movement.

The brain stem is a bundle of nerve fibers and a combination of organs in the center of the head, near the place where the skull and the spine meet. It has a number of functions, including the regulation of heartbeat, breathing, and blood pressure. It is primarily known as the message relay center of the brain, and it delivers information from the body to the brain and sends commands from the brain to the body. When sensations such as heat, cold, or pain are present, the messages are sent along nerve fibers to the brain, passing through the brain stem on the way. The brain receives the message and understands that part of the body is too warm, too cold, or experiencing pain.

Sensory information—such as sights, sounds, and tastes—also passes through the brain stem. This allows the brain to interpret the incoming information. The brain stem also transfers orders from the brain to the body. When a person moves or speaks, the commands to do so are initiated in the brain and sent through the brain stem to the muscles.

The brain is fragile, so it is protected by a thick covering called the meninges. The meninges are made up of three layers: a thick, tough outer covering called the dura mater; a thin, flexible bottom layer called the pia mater, which contains many blood vessels; and a middle layer called the arachnoid that is made up of netlike tissue filled with fluid. The meninges help cushion the brain against impact to the head. This is the place where migraine pain is generally felt because the brain itself has no pain receptors.

The thalamus is a brain structure that is important in understanding migraines. It is a small structure at the top of the brain stem. It receives all sensory impulses for sight, sound, touch, and taste, but it does not receive information for the sense of smell. The thalamus relays the incoming information to the appropriate parts of the cerebrum.

In order to function normally, human brains depend on a number of chemicals. These chemicals keep the brain healthy, assist in the transmission of messages, and maintain mood. One of the most important brain chemicals is serotonin; in addition to regulating mood, one of its jobs is to help regulate pain messages traveling through the brain stem. Serotonin is a chemical messenger that transmits nerve signals between nerve cells and also causes blood vessels to narrow. Serotonin is believed to play a part in migraines.

Theories About Migraines

Researchers have not yet identified the causes and the progression of a migraine inside the head. Past theories proposed that blood vessels inside the head became constricted, causing warning signs, and that the blood vessels then dilated, causing the headache pain. Current theories indicate that this is only partly true; although changes in blood flow do not cause the pain, researchers believe they may make it worse.

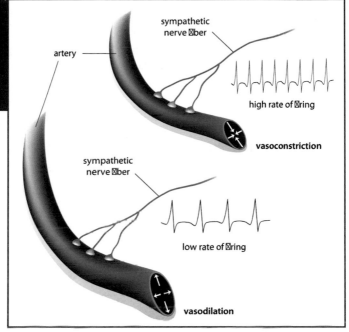

Migraine pain is made worse by constriction and dilation of blood vessels.

sympathetic nerve fiber

artery

high rate of firing

vasoconstriction

sympathetic nerve fiber

low rate of firing

vasodilation

In current research, doctors are considering several different theories of how a migraine gets started. New theories regard migraines as too complex to be caused only by changes in blood vessels. One theory, called cortical spreading depression (CSD), proposes that the neurons, or brain cells, of migraine patients are easily excited. When a migraine is triggered, the neurons suddenly fire electrical pulses that ripple across the brain in a wave. The ripple travels down the brain stem, where pain centers are located. This ripple causes blood flow to increase sharply and then drop off quickly. The actual pain is caused by the changes in blood vessels, stimulation in the brain stem, or both. However, the way migraines react to a form of treatment called transcranial magnetic stimulation (tTMS) has made some researchers doubt that CSD is a migraine cause.

Another theory about migraines suggests that the trigeminal nerve, a major nerve inside the head, plays a role in migraine pain. The theory is that the trigeminal nerve fires between migraine attacks and in turn stimulates arteries in the scalp and the meninges. When the trigeminal nerve is malfunctioning, it creates problems in the way the brain interprets stimuli, so a migraine may be a brain's overreaction to a certain stimulus that would not cause pain in someone with a properly functioning trigeminal nerve. This malfunction activates nerve fibers that send pain impulses. The nearby blood vessels dilate, and inflammation is caused in the surrounding tissues, also causing pain. Brain chemicals involved in these processes may sensitize nearby nerve endings, which makes them more likely than usual to fire off pain messages. All of these pain messages then travel to the cerebrum, which tells the patient they are getting a migraine. This theory also accounts for why there are so many different types of migraine pain. Starting in the brain stem, the nerve spreads out across the front of the head and face, affecting many different parts. As writer Tammy Rome explained on Migraine.com, "One person will feel pain in and around the eye. Another will feel pain in the face and cheeks ... Yet another will complain of phantom tooth pain. Sometimes the forehead, or temple, or even the ears hurt."[4] The part that hurts depends on which part of the trigeminal nerve is sending faulty pain signals.

Current migraine theory also suggests that brain chemicals play a role. Doctors believe excitable brain cells trigger a release of brain chemicals such as serotonin, causing constriction in blood vessels and a reduction

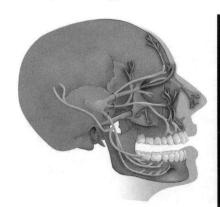

The trigeminal nerve originates in the brain and spreads throughout the head and face. This weblike nerve is shown here.

in blood flow around the brain. Then, serotonin drops to a level that is extremely low. When serotonin levels decrease, the blood vessels dilate and cause migraine pain. The chemical estrogen may also play a role for women.

Doctors admit that no single, definitive theory of migraines exists. They acknowledge that a migraine might be caused by a combination of the factors described above, and the exact mechanism of a migraine might be different in different patients. Further study will bring researchers closer to a true understanding of migraines and allow a greater chance of a cure for these headaches.

When to See a Doctor

A person should see a doctor or visit an emergency room as quickly as possible if any of the following situations occur. These can be signs of a life-threatening condition.

- A headache is sudden and extremely severe.

- A headache follows a blow to the head.

- Confusion or drowsiness occurs along with a headache.

- A headache comes with numbness, double or blurred vision, slurred speech, or the inability to speak.

- Lack of coordination accompanies a headache.

- The headache sufferer also experiences weakness on one side of the body.

- Severe vomiting or seizures take place with the headache.

- A headache comes with a high fever, neck pain, sore muscles or joints, jaw pain, or vision loss.

Getting a Diagnosis

Many people who suffer from headaches relieve their pain by using OTC medicines such as aspirin, ibuprofen, or acetaminophen. These can be purchased without a doctor's prescription. When pain is so intense that these medicines have little effect or when a patient's headaches are frequent, a diagnosis by a doctor is needed to determine the type of headache so proper treatment can be given.

Depending on a patient's symptoms, a doctor might quickly suspect that the patient suffers from migraines. However, some headaches, including migraines, are not easy to classify. In those cases, a doctor will also look for simple causes of headaches, such as flu, colds, allergies, or dehydration. A doctor can quickly recognize symptoms of certain diseases, such as meningitis, and confirm or rule out such illnesses. If those ailments are not present, more information is needed to classify a patient's headache.

Doctors typically take a patient's medical history. They ask questions about a patient's past illnesses, accidents, or injuries. They also ask whether a patient's family members suffer from headaches because some headaches, especially migraines, tend to run in families. A doctor will want to hear a precise description of the patient's headaches, including the length of the headaches and the type of pain. Headaches can be described in many different ways—some of the descriptions include stabbing, pounding, throbbing, dull, sharp, aching, stinging, shooting, pressure, and pins and needles. Sometimes the type of pain can help a doctor recognize the nature of the headache.

If the cause of a patient's headache is still uncertain, a doctor might order medical tests. These tests will help a doctor identify things that are not causing the

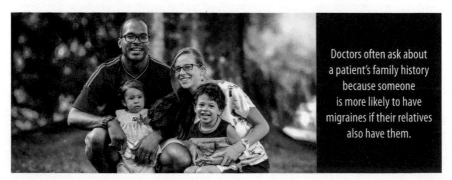

Doctors often ask about a patient's family history because someone is more likely to have migraines if their relatives also have them.

pain and rule out secondary headaches. Some of the tests that might be used include:

- A blood test, in which blood is drawn from the patient and examined in a laboratory. This can rule out an infection.
- X-rays, such as those used to examine broken bones, which can identify defects or abnormalities of the skull, jaw, teeth, or neck. Unusual formations or alignment in the bones or teeth could cause pain.
- Magnetic resonance imaging (MRI), a painless test that uses magnets to create an image of the inside of the body. MRI tests might reveal or rule out conditions such as a stroke, an aneurysm, a tumor, or brain abnormalities, and they can also examine the blood vessels in the brain to find anything unusual.
- A computerized tomography (CT) or computerized axial tomography (CAT) scan, another painless test that produces images of the inside of the body. It can detect problems such as infections, skull fractures, sinus diseases, bleeding in the brain (hemorrhage), and tumors.

Not all of these tests are necessary for everyone who has a headache. Sometimes headaches fit the pattern of a migraine so closely that doctors immediately recognize them as migraines without any tests. When tests are needed, doctors generally ask for one test at a time, examine the results, and then decide whether more tests are necessary.

If a doctor fails to find a sign of a disease after running all of these tests, then it is possible that the headaches are migraines. No single test currently exists to identify a migraine. When a diagnosis is made that a patient suffers from migraines, it is based on ruling out other causes and then matching the headaches to the typical symptoms and patterns of migraines.

Migraines and Biological Sex

Biological sex plays a role in how people experience pain, including headaches. About 18 percent of women—compared with only 6 percent of men—experience migraines. Experts agree this is partially due to hormones; about 60 percent of women who get migraines find that their attacks are related to the hormonal changes that accompany their menstrual cycle. Other research suggests women may be more sensitive to things that trigger migraines than men or are sensitive to different things. For instance, women are more likely to get migraines in response to changing weather patterns, while men are more likely to get them during physical activity. Alcohol triggers migraines in both sexes, but since men tend to drink more, they report it as a migraine trigger more frequently.

Additionally, among migraine sufferers, women are likely to report higher levels of pain than men. In addition to being another effect of hormones, recent research suggests it may be partially due to differences in the brains of male and female migraine sufferers. In a 2012 study, brain scans found that the gray matter that makes up the brain was thicker in two parts of a female migraine sufferer's brain: the posterior insula, which plays a role in pain processing, and the precuneus, where some researchers believe a person's sense of self may be located. According to *Science* magazine, "In women with migraines, 'these thicker areas talk to each other and work together to respond to pain' in a pattern not seen in the men, [lead researcher Nasim] Maleki says."[1] Further research must be done to confirm these results, but they may lead to differences in the ways migraines are treated between men and women.

1. Carol Cruzan Morton, "Why Do Women Get More Migraines?," *Science*, August 13, 2012. www.sciencemag.org/news/2012/08/why-do-women-get-more-migraines.

Different Kinds of Migraines

Migraines can vary widely from one patient to another and even from one headache to another in the same patient. However, all migraines meet a set of criteria established by the International Headache Society in 1988 and revised in 2013. According to its standards, a headache is a migraine if it shows the following characteristics:

1. The patient has had at least five similar headaches.
2. The headache lasts from four to seventy-two hours if it is not treated or if treatment does not work.

3. The patient has at least two of the following symptoms:
    a. pain on only one side of the head (unilateral pain)
    b. a pulsing or throbbing sensation
    c. moderate to severe pain that prevents the patient from fully taking part in daily activities
    d. the headache gets worse during physical activity, such as climbing stairs or bending over
4. The headache comes with one of the following conditions:
    a. nausea or vomiting
    b. lights and noises make the patient uncomfortable, and the patient seeks out a dark, quiet place
5. A secondary headache is ruled out through a doctor's exam or medical tests.

One of the first steps a doctor will take in diagnosing a headache is to compare a patient's symptoms with this list. If the symptoms match the list exactly, the doctor will know the headache is a migraine. The doctor and the patient can then work together to understand the migraines and find ways to manage them.

Although these criteria cover all migraines, there are different kinds of migraines a person can be diagnosed with. Each one comes with a different set of symptoms. Getting a correct diagnosis determines the appropriate treatment. The wide range of migraine symptoms makes this disorder especially interesting and challenging to doctors and researchers. As painful and disabling as migraines are, their fascinating and unusual symptoms raise many questions about exactly what goes on in the human brain.

CHAPTER TWO

DIFFERENCES AMONG MIGRAINES

With so many different kinds of migraines, it is clear that not everyone experiences them the same way. This is important to recognize because some people may be accused of faking a migraine if their symptoms are not the same as another migraine sufferer. Even people who get the same kind of migraines may have different symptoms. Getting an accurate diagnosis and recognizing their personal triggers can help people with migraines gain more control over their condition.

Examining Genes

Doctors and patients have known for years that a tendency for migraines can be passed from parent to child. Statistics show that 70 to 75 percent of migraine patients have at least one relative in their immediate family who also suffers from migraines, and children have a higher risk of developing migraines if one or both parents get them. When patients understand their family history of migraines, this can help diagnose and manage their pain.

Most migraines are polygenic, meaning more than one gene is responsible. A gene is a unit of information that gets passed down from parent to child. Almost every cell in the body contains chromosomes, which are long strings of genes that are coiled up into packages and are responsible for everything about a person: eye color, number of fingers, any diseases or disorders, and so on. Polygenic traits and disorders involve several different genes working together; monogenic traits and disorders, which are rarer, involve a mutation, or change, in just one gene.

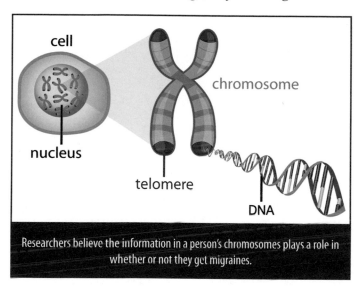

cell

nucleus

chromosome

telomere

DNA

Researchers believe the information in a person's chromosomes plays a role in whether or not they get migraines.

In 2008, the results of a study seeking a genetic link for migraines were published in Europe. Researchers worked with more than 1,700 international patients to find a genetic similarity among families. The project discovered a gene that is believed to carry the migraine tendency. Researchers Aarno Palotie and Verneri Anttila were excited. They announced, "This study is the first international collaboration as well as the largest linkage study in migraine [disease] to date. It successfully applied new analysis strategies ... and paved the way for more large studies."[5] As of 2017, a total of four genes have been found to play a role in what is now called familial hemiplegic migraine (FHM). It is divided into three types: For instance, FHM1 means there is a mutation on the CACNA1A gene. Only three of the four genes are considered when making a diagnosis because researchers are still unsure exactly how the fourth gene causes migraines.

FHM is extremely rare, affecting only 0.01 percent of the population. It causes numbness or temporary paralysis on one side of the body ("hemi" means half and "plegic" means paralysis) as well as dizziness and sometimes difficulty seeing or speaking.

Migraine Classifications

There is much confusion around the topic of migraine classification and diagnosis. Some terms are generally used only by medical professionals, and sometimes people confuse similar types of migraines. The official guideline is called the International Classification of Headache Disorders (ICHD), currently in its third edition. However, people who are familiar with the older terms may still use them. Additionally, most people who get migraines do not have access to the ICHD-III, so they may get their information from online sources that have not been updated.

As previously mentioned, migraine without aura—previously called common migraine—is the type most people experience. This or migraine with aura—previously called classic, complex, or complicated migraine—is what most people think of when they think of a migraine. The symptoms are similar; the only difference is the aura.

An ocular migraine is a term that is used to describe any migraine that causes vision changes. This can include migraine with aura as well as a retinal migraine, which "is a rare condition occurring in a person who has experienced other symptoms of migraine."[6] While migraine with aura generally affects both eyes, a retinal migraine affects only one and "involves repeated bouts of short-lasting, diminished vision or blindness. These bouts may precede or accompany a headache."[7] According to the Mayo Clinic, loss of vision in one eye is generally caused by something more serious than a migraine and is cause for a trip to the doctor.

Migraine equivalent, migraine without headache, or typical aura without headache are all names for a type of migraine that can be recognized by all the symptoms of a migraine except pain. Because the pain is absent, many people who experience one do not realize they have a migraine. Even though they are not painful, they can still make it difficult for the person to do typical activities because of the nausea and vision changes they experience. Sometimes the aura involves stroke-like symptoms, as previously mentioned.

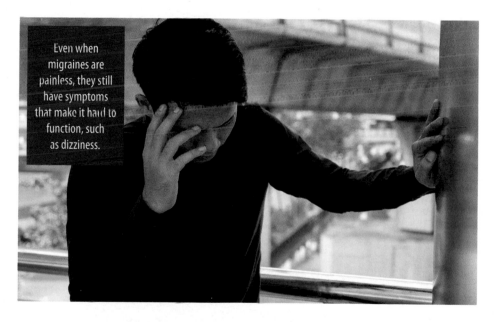

Even when migraines are painless, they still have symptoms that make it hard to function, such as dizziness.

Migraine with brain stem aura, formerly called basilar-type migraine, is a type of migraine that most often affects children and young adults. It is a type of migraine with aura where the symptoms come from the brain stem; they include problems seeing, dizziness, loss of balance, poor muscle control, slurred speech, ringing in the ears, and fainting. The headache pain is generally felt on both sides of the head, rather than only one as is typical with other types of migraine. Teenage girls are the most common sufferers, and it is often linked to their menstrual cycle.

Other conditions that were previously considered migraines have been dropped from the ICHD-III. This does not mean they are not still real and serious conditions, just that they are no longer officially considered migraines. According to Dr. Peter Goadsby, "one of the top doctors influencing IHS and AHS policies ... the World Health Organization needed a common language to define all the Migraine subtypes so that doctors and patients around the world could compare notes and exchange data."[8] However, the word "migraine" is generally still applied to some of these conditions—even by some medical professionals—although some of them are only complications of migraines. They include:

- *Abdominal migraine*: vomiting and dizziness without a headache that occurs at irregular intervals. It is most common in children. If the pattern of attacks is predictable, it is called cyclical vomiting. Most children who experience abdominal migraine will develop migraine headaches when they get older.
- *Hormonal or menstrual migraine*: as the name suggests, migraines that appear or are made worse when a woman gets her period.
- *Morning migraine*: migraine-like symptoms that are present upon waking up.
- *Weather-related migraine*: migraine-like symptoms that are linked to changes in the weather.
- *Migralepsy*: a rare complication in which a migraine with aura triggers a seizure. It is also called migraine aura-triggered seizure.
- *Vestibular migraine*: "a nervous system problem that causes repeated dizziness (or vertigo) in people who have a history of migraine symptoms."[9] It may also be called migraine-associated vertigo, migrainous

vertigo, or migraine-related vestibulopathy.

- *Status migraine*: a migraine that lasts more than 72 hours. It is considered a medical emergency because in rare cases, it can cause a stroke.

Myths versus Reality

Anyone who has ever had a true migraine can attest that the pain and other symptoms, such as nausea and dizziness, are very real and difficult to deal with. However, many people who suffer from migraines are misunderstood. Some people think they are simply overly dramatic. Others may think the person is just lazy and using the migraine as an excuse to get out of work. Women with migraines are more likely than men to be treated as attention-seeking because of gender stereotypes in Western society: Complaining about pain is seen as a feminine trait, while bearing it quietly is seen as a masculine one. For this reason, some people believe that if a man speaks up about his pain, it must be truly unbearable, while a woman who speaks up about her pain may be seen as overly sensitive. A theory that was popular in the early 20th century was that there was a "migraine personality"—a particular set of personality traits that made people more likely to get a migraine. These included "high-strung, perfectionist, anxious worriers"[10] and went along with stereotypes about women and their perceived lack of ability to handle stress. This myth has persisted through the 21st century, and even though it has been disproven, some people—even some doctors—still believe in it. Writer Anna Eidt explained the problem with this way of thinking:

> *Despite research that shows our personality traits are not fixed and can actually ... shift significantly in reaction to our environments and relationships, generally we tend to think of our personalities as a fixed set of characteristics ... Believing that ...*

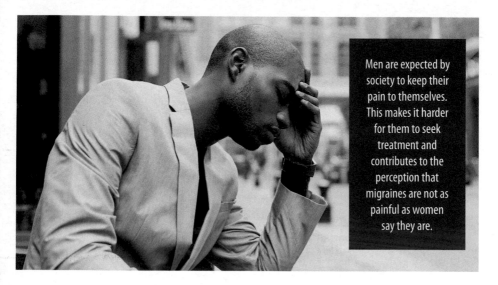

Men are expected by society to keep their pain to themselves. This makes it harder for them to seek treatment and contributes to the perception that migraines are not as painful as women say they are.

migraine is somehow intrinsically [naturally] a part of who we are can lead to shame, hopelessness, and self-blame on top of the already difficult mix of emotions involved in living with disabling migraine attacks, and that's just not helpful.[11]

Although stress can be a contributing factor in migraine attacks, it is not the only one, and dismissing migraines as a simple problem with stress management can prevent people from getting the treatment they need.

Because migraines occur with such a wide range of symptoms, they often go unrecognized, and a patient may not even realize they are experiencing migraines, especially if they occur without pain. A person's family and coworkers often do not understand what a migraine is about, especially if the patient's symptoms are outside of what is recognized as the "typical" migraine. Someone who reports nausea and an aura or an intense headache but no other symptoms may falsely be accused of lying about having a migraine by people who believe all migraines are the same. Even doctors sometimes have difficulty diagnosing migraines. To make matters more difficult, no medical testing exists that can prove that a person has a migraine. This confusing set of circumstances can bring about anxiety for the person with the migraine, making them feel that they must explain themselves to others or keep quiet about it completely.

What Not to Say

People who do not experience migraines often say things to their loved ones or even to strangers that come off as offensive. The person may be trying to help, but some things are generally not helpful for a migraine sufferer to hear, including:

- "It's just a headache."
- "I know how you feel; I get headaches sometimes, too."
- "Move around/distract yourself, and you'll feel better."
- "You should stop [common trigger]."
- "You don't look sick."
- "You should try [treatment]."
- "At least it's not [life-threatening illness]."
- "It'll get better eventually."
- "You need to manage stress better."
- "I thought only women get migraines."
- "I wish I could stay home from work/school like you do."

Although scientists do not know exactly how migraines are caused, they do know they are due to biological and chemical changes in the brain; they are not something a person can control. Everyone's body and migraines are different, and what works for one person might not work for another. People who get migraines generally do not appreciate getting medical advice from anyone other than their doctor; they know what works and does not work for them. Additionally, hearing that other people are worse off does not make someone feel better when they are suffering at that moment. People can support a loved one with migraines by being caring and understanding—for example, by leaving someone alone when they are having an attack.

Identifying Triggers

Researchers have identified more than a dozen different possible migraine triggers, or things that bring on a migraine attack. These triggers are different among different people and can even vary from one headache to the next. Stress might bring on a migraine in someone at one point, but weather or motion sickness might start a migraine at a different time. This variety of triggers is another reason why understanding migraines is sometimes tricky.

Neurologist and professor Richard Lipton of the Albert Einstein College of Medicine at Yeshiva University believes every patient must make an effort to understand their own migraines: "Education and empowerment are the keys to successful Migraine management. Patients who understand their disease, identify their triggers, and learn to use both behavioral strategies and medications effectively can dramatically reduce their burden of illness."[12]

One of the most common migraine triggers is stress. Stress can come from many sources—pressure at work or school, trouble in a marriage or other relationship, the death of a loved one, or the day-to-day pressure of always being on the go.

Researchers divide stress into two types. The first type is the stress of a life-changing event, such as a death, divorce, job change, or move to a new place. When these events cause a migraine, the migraine typically occurs as the event is nearing a conclusion—for example, after a funeral is over or a move has been completed. These migraines are sometimes called letdown migraines because they occur as a person is beginning to relax from extreme stress.

The second type of stress is the kind that comes with the daily pressure of work and family. After days or weeks of job demands, carpools, making meals, and other expectations, the built-up stress may trigger a migraine. In children or teens, the routine of school and homework plus the pressure of sports or other activities, a part-time job or babysitting, and household chores may contribute to triggering a migraine. It is important to remember that not everyone gets stressed by the same things, so loved ones should be understanding and compassionate when someone tells them they are experiencing stress, even if it is from something the person does not find stressful themselves.

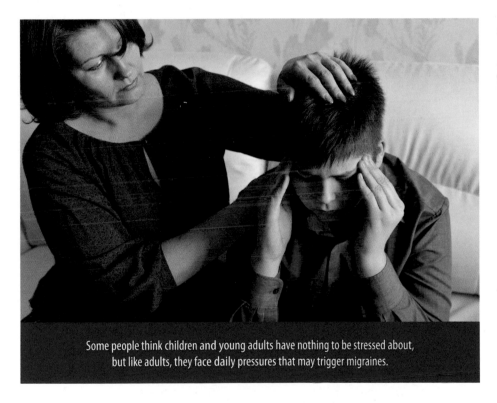

Some people think children and young adults have nothing to be stressed about, but like adults, they face daily pressures that may trigger migraines.

Getting too much or too little sleep is known to trigger migraines in some people. These people find that staying on a regular schedule and getting about the same amount of sleep each night can reduce the chance of triggering a sleep-related migraine.

In the same way that loud noises and bright lights can become painful during the headache phase of a migraine, some people report that lights or sounds can actually trigger a migraine. Loud music, traffic noise, machinery, car horns, or even the sounds of a large crowd at a shopping mall or stadium have been known to trigger migraines. Bright lights—such as streetlights or car lights at night, lightning, or camera flashes—can be migraine triggers. Sunlight, especially when reflected off snow, roads, or water, is another trigger. Sunglasses are effective at cutting glare and reducing the chance of a migraine. Some migraine sufferers take precautions by wearing sunglasses or ear plugs if they suspect they will encounter conditions that could trigger a headache. Looking at a computer screen for a long time can also be a migraine trigger. Turning the brightness down on the computer monitor may help.

Not Just an Adult Problem

Migraines might seem like an adult disorder, but they also affect a large number of children. Children as young as five have been diagnosed with recurring migraines. One out of about 20 children (roughly 8 million in the United States) has experienced a migraine. Up until the age of 10, boys and girls get migraines at about an equal rate. After puberty, however, the numbers of girls with migraines far surpasses the boys—girls get about three times as many migraines.

During the high school years, approximately 20 percent of students will get a migraine. These numbers decrease for boys in this age group but increase for girls. Some students report that they get two to three migraines per week.

Migraines in children tend to be shorter, lasting one to forty-eight hours. The pain tends to be all over the head rather than the one-sided pain that is common in adults. Drinking plenty of water and getting enough sleep are recommended to help children avoid migraines. Parents are also advised to monitor the consumption of trigger foods and watch for any related migraine episodes.

Head injuries often produce headache pain, and they can also trigger a migraine. A blow to the head—such as a sports injury or car crash—is capable of starting a migraine, sometimes within minutes of the accident. Neck trauma, including whiplash,

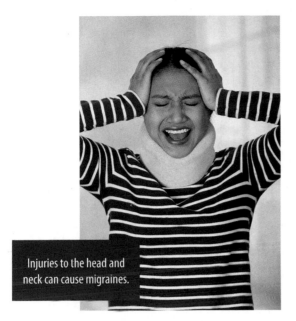

Injuries to the head and neck can cause migraines.

which is caused by an abrupt stop or impact, is also sometimes a migraine trigger, even in people who have never had a migraine before. In some people, a less severe headache can turn into a migraine if it is left untreated, even if no head or neck injury has occurred. For example, someone may wake up with a mild headache due to not getting enough sleep. In most people, this headache will go away on its own after awhile, especially if the person is able to take a nap, but for some people, the headache will get steadily worse until it is a migraine. People who experience this issue can generally avoid the migraine by taking OTC pain medication before the headache gets worse.

More than three-quarters of migraine sufferers report that changes in weather can bring about a migraine. This may include the movement of a warm or cold front, thunderstorms, extremely high or low humidity, or an abrupt drop in atmospheric pressure.

Just as some people can become highly sensitive to strong smells during the headache phase of a migraine, certain odors are also known to trigger migraines. These are smells such as car exhaust, tobacco smoke, perfumes and aftershaves, paint, and chemicals. The effect of these smells is worse in a confined space, such as an airplane, an elevator, or a room with closed doors.

Research shows that migraine sufferers are also

more prone to motion sickness than are people who do not get migraines. Evidence also suggests that adults who experience migraines likely suffered from motion sickness in childhood. The connection between motion sickness and migraines is not understood. Motion sickness also appears to be a migraine trigger for some people.

Hormones are natural chemicals produced by the body to regulate a variety of functions, including growth, puberty, pregnancy, and menopause. Changes in hormone levels are known to cause migraines. Women go through a cycle of hormone levels every month, and their hormones change dramatically during pregnancy. Many women report that their migraines are brought on at certain times of the month or during or after pregnancy. Migraine patient Marilyn Hartman knew her migraines were linked to hormones because they improved after she went through menopause and her hormone activity decreased: "I got my first migraine when I was thirty-five years old. After that, I had a headache every day for sixteen years, with a migraine once or twice a week. After I reached menopause, the migraines mostly went away. I'm still sensitive to bright light and glare, especially bright sun on the snow in winter."[13]

The list of migraine triggers is long. Some triggers are very common, but certain others are rare or unusual. Some less common triggers are fluorescent lighting, certain prescription medications, strenuous exercise, smoking, secondhand smoke, and combined environmental factors such as air-conditioning, office or industrial machinery, and plastic or vinyl smells. For some people, these individual triggers do not cause migraines, but specific combinations may set off the headache. For example, air-conditioning might not start a headache, but the combination of air-conditioning, fluorescent lighting, and machinery noises might bring on a migraine.

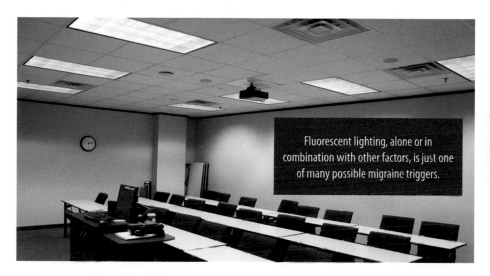

Fluorescent lighting, alone or in combination with other factors, is just one of many possible migraine triggers.

Certain foods are also common triggers. Many people who experience migraines see a concrete link between foods that contain tyramine—a natural compound in foods that is known to cause blood vessels to dilate—and the onset of a migraine. Researchers have noted this link but are unsure of the exact role tyramine plays. Some believe high levels of tyramine can trigger the release of other migraine-causing brain chemicals. Tyramine tends to appear in foods that are aged, such as certain cheeses, and liquids that are brewed, such as beer and soy sauce. Salami and sauerkraut are especially high in tyramine. However, not every food that triggers a migraine contains tyramine, and food triggers can be different for everyone. Common food triggers include:

- aged cheeses, such as sharp cheddar or blue cheese
- alcoholic beverages, especially beer and red wine
- aspartame (an artificial sweetener found in diet

soda and other foods)
- caffeine
- chocolate
- MSG (monosodium glutamate, a food preservative and flavor enhancer)
- sulfites (preservatives often used in dried fruits or wine)
- sodium nitrate and sodium nitrite (food preservatives found in hot dogs, lunch meat, and sausage)

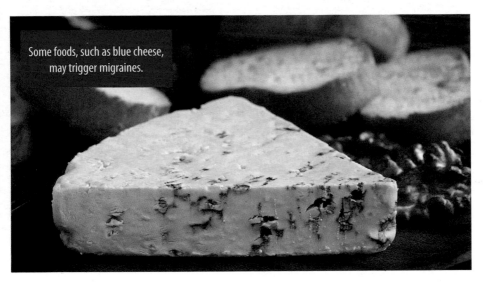

Some foods, such as blue cheese, may trigger migraines.

In the category of food triggers, caffeine and chocolate deserve special mention. Whereas some people report that these are migraine triggers, others crave these foods during migraines. Still others say caffeine or chocolate actually help calm down the headache; some people can avoid taking medication if they drink a cup of coffee or a caffeinated energy drink, either every day or only when they feel a migraine coming on. Caffeine is a common ingredient in some OTC headache and migraine pain relievers. People prone to migraines are wise to pay attention to the effects of these substances and add or subtract them from their diets to better manage their migraines.

More unusually, some foods become triggers only when in combination with other foods. Migraine patient Nancy Mildebrandt has to avoid chocolate and cheese on the same day. She explained, "I can eat chocolate without problems, and I can eat cheese. But if I eat one of them, and then eat the other on the same day, I'm almost certain to get a migraine."[14]

For those suffering from migraines, discovering triggers is like striking gold. Each time they identify a new trigger, they have a greater ability to manage their migraines. By avoiding these triggers, they can greatly reduce the number of headaches that occur or be prepared for headaches once they start. Every migraine is a learning process; people who experience migraines continually analyze their lives and their headaches to discover ways to reduce the impact of migraines.

CHAPTER THREE

MANAGING MIGRAINES

Although medications for general pain and for migraines in particular do exist, migraines still require management. Avoiding a migraine is the best course of action because many medications take some time to start working, and sometimes they do not work at all if they are taken too late or if the migraine is more painful than usual. Some migraines force a person to stay in bed, but others might allow them to struggle through the day. Either way, the headaches can disrupt or ruin a person's day.

Migraines are difficult to live with and complex to understand. However, when people analyze their migraines and make an effort to understand them, they take a huge step toward minimizing the amount of time that they suffer. Doctors and patients have discovered a number of ways to recognize, identify, and shorten migraine episodes.

Tracking Migraines

Although there are some common migraine triggers, not every person who experiences migraines shares the same triggers. In fact, sometimes triggers are not even consistent for one person. For example, if one of someone's triggers is red wine, they may be able to sometimes have a glass of red wine without experiencing a migraine. However, people with inconsistent triggers generally avoid the trigger completely because to them, taking the chance on a glass of red wine or some other kind of food is not worth the risk that they may end up with a migraine. Over time, most migraine sufferers learn to recognize at least some of their triggers.

Some triggers, such as a certain food, smoking, lack of sleep, or loud music can be relatively easy to manage. Avoiding these triggers might be inconvenient at times—skipping pizza or avoiding public places with loud music might not seem like much fun—but the alternative of a full-blown migraine is far worse. Doctors recommend that migraine patients make an effort to understand and avoid their triggers.

Other triggers cannot be avoided, such as hormones, changes in the weather, or the noises and smells associated with traffic. People who have these triggers might carry medication with them so they can begin treatment if they suspect the beginning of a migraine.

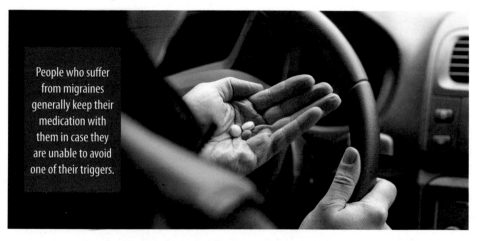

People who suffer from migraines generally keep their medication with them in case they are unable to avoid one of their triggers.

Patterns can be hard to recognize; for example, someone may notice that they sometimes get a migraine after eating cheese and assume that is one of their triggers, while ignoring the fact that on the days they ate cheese, they also did not get much sleep the night before. For this reason, many doctors recommend that migraine patients keep a journal so patterns are easier to spot. In the journal, they record all the foods they eat, their activities, and any unusual symptoms they may feel. Any symptom, no matter how minor, can be important. Feelings of tiredness, depression, weakness, or dizziness can all be warning symptoms, although many people may brush them off as unimportant.

When a migraine occurs, patients record all of the symptoms and any medications they take. They also record any factors that make the headache better or worse. Then, when a migraine is over, a patient can look back at the journal and try to detect any triggers or warning signs. After several migraines, patients might discover a pattern—for example, that they ate a certain food, got stuck in traffic on a hot day, or experienced a high level of stress. Because changes in weather can be a factor in migraines, weather conditions should also be recorded in the journal.

Migraine patient Wayne Hoffmann discovered patterns in his migraines:

> *I didn't get migraines very often, but when I did, they put me in bed for two days. I figured out that they hit me after major stressful events. Then I read an article about food triggers and realized that red wine and blue cheese would cause headaches for me. It was easy to avoid those foods after that, and it cut down on the number of migraines I would get.*[15]

Keeping a journal to identify triggers is an important part of helping a patient manage their migraines and can show some surprising trends. In a 2016 study, researchers analyzed the migraine journals that 284 participants kept over 90 days. They found that some things people thought were triggers actually had nothing to do with their migraines, and more surprisingly, that some things commonly seen as triggers could actually protect against migraines. For example, the researchers found that while travel can be a migraine trigger for some people because of the stress involved, for others it can be protective because a long trip on a plane or bus can give them a chance to relax. As Dr. Stephen Donoghue, one of the researchers in this study, said, "So it may be that relaxation is the 'true' protector ... We are careful to tell people that they need to think about the context in which the 'protector' occurs."[16]

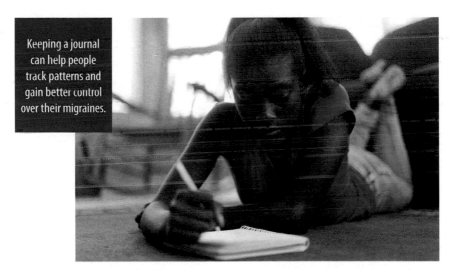

Keeping a journal can help people track patterns and gain better control over their migraines.

The study also revealed that most people's migraines are unique to them, which makes it even more important for people to track their own triggers and protective factors. If people know what they should avoid or seek out, they will feel less helpless when it comes to preventing migraines.

Using a Visual Aid

Another effective way to evaluate and record headaches is to draw a map or picture. Describing the location and type of pain to a doctor can be difficult, especially for children. Remembering what the pain was like after a few weeks or months can also be hard. When each headache is a little different, this process can be even more complicated. Making sketches of headaches can be a valuable tool in understanding them. The picture could be of the face, the top or back of the head, the side of the head, or all of these angles, depending on the type of headache. Jagged or wiggly lines, colors, or drawings of hammers or lightning bolts might be used to represent the type and location of pain. Artistry is not important, but the record of the headache is valuable in determining how to treat migraines.

Unusual Pain Triggers

The medical definition of allodynia is "pain from stimuli which are not normally painful."[1] Allodynia sometimes comes with a migraine. People prone to migraines have reported several types of allodynia, including the following:

- sensitive scalp

- sore muscles on head or neck

- pain while combing hair

- pain from cold air contacting the head

- a headache worsened by heat from a hair dryer, stove, or fireplace

- discomfort from wearing clothes

- pain from wearing jewelry

When allodynia occurs, a migraine is generally in full swing. The appearance of allodynia is often a sign that the migraine is so far along that medication will be unable to prevent it. This is why paying attention to early warning signs is important.

1. "Definition of Allodynia," MedicineNet.com. www.medicinenet.com/script/main/art.asp?articlekey=25197.

Paying Attention to the Signals

Even when a person makes every effort to control their lifestyle, migraines can still take hold. Many people report good success in avoiding a migraine if they take steps as soon as they recognize a warning signal. This might mean taking medication, grabbing a quick nap, or finding a dark, quiet place for a break.

During Super Bowl XXXII in 1998, Denver

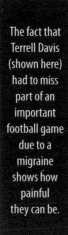

The fact that Terrell Davis (shown here) had to miss part of an important football game due to a migraine shows how painful they can be.

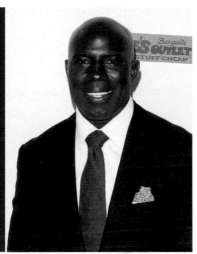

Broncos running back and current NFL Hall of Famer Terrell Davis recognized his oncoming migraine. "In all the games I've ever played in my life, it had to come on this Sunday. I noticed I had a headache ... I couldn't see."[17] He left the game to take his medication, missed the second quarter, and returned to the game after halftime. Davis's medication succeeded in blocking the migraine. He scored three touchdowns in the game and was voted Most Valuable Player. The Denver Broncos defeated the Green Bay Packers to win the Super Bowl.

Not all migraines are blocked with this level of success, but early intervention can make all the difference in avoiding an episode. Many migraine sufferers report that taking medication at the first warning sign is the key to getting relief, especially since some migraine medications will only work if they are taken before the attack starts.

Day-to-Day Life

Some people who experience migraines feel that the worst part of a migraine is not the pain but the effect it has on everyday life. Migraines frequently cause a person to miss work or school and then have to catch up when the migraine is over. Migraine episodes can also interfere with sports, social activities, housework, vacations, and special occasions such as weddings and graduations. With no reliable method to predict when a migraine will hit, migraine sufferers are sometimes at the mercy of their own bodies.

When migraines cause people to miss work, they either lose out on wages or their employer gives them sick pay. People with chronic migraines generally miss more days of work than people with episodic migraines, but lost work time includes days when the migraine patient was at work but had difficulty functioning normally and was not working at full efficiency. Some people who do not receive sick pay from their job force themselves to go to work out of fear that they will be fired if they miss too many days.

Lost wages are only part of the picture. Migraine patients also suffer anxiety from missing work. They worry that missing work or low productivity could result in getting fired or being passed up for promotions or raises. They worry about what coworkers think of their illness; some people simply do not understand or do not believe that migraines are real. Migraine patients who do not get a lot done at work on days when they are feeling sick may be unfairly seen as lazy. This anxiety can cause stress that contributes to more migraines.

Migraine sufferers also feel an impact on their social lives. Some are unable to attend activities with friends if known triggers will be present, such as odors, noises, or bright lights. Shopping, concerts, and sporting events might present strong migraine triggers and require someone prone to migraines to stay away. The possible onset of a migraine could cause someone to cancel plans for a movie, dinner, or other social activity.

Guilt is a common emotion in migraine sufferers when they miss out on activities, fall behind at work, or do not accomplish household tasks. Even though they know that their condition is real, and they know firsthand the severity of their pain, they still suffer from guilt at times over a physical condition that they cannot control. This is why it is not helpful for loved ones to remind them of how much they have missed due to their migraines. Migraine patients would prefer to keep their headaches under control, but sometimes this is simply not possible.

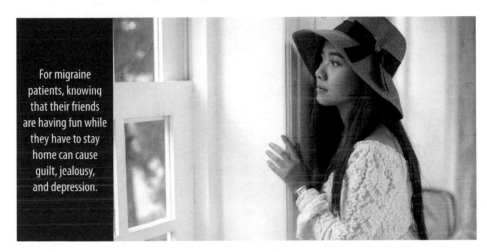

For migraine patients, knowing that their friends are having fun while they have to stay home can cause guilt, jealousy, and depression.

Migraine sufferers are often the targets of bad advice. This might come from a well-meaning friend or relative or an insensitive stranger or coworker. Most of the time, bad advice comes from someone who does not understand migraines or who believes a migraine is just a simple headache. Migraine sufferers might hear things such as, "Just walk it off," "Take more pain medicine," "Try to push through it," or "You're just being dramatic." Statements such as these do not help the person and tend to cause more anxiety and guilt.

Emotional Effects

For many years, doctors have suspected a link between migraines and mild mental illness. Bouts of depression and anxiety were recognized as signals in the warning phase in some patients. Theories were posed that some migraine patients suffered from these emotional effects as a result of migraine pain or as a side effect of missing out on events, continually catching up, and the guilt of not accomplishing daily tasks.

Studies have shown that migraine sufferers are two to five times more likely than nonsufferers to experience depression and anxiety. According to the American Migraine Foundation, about 25 percent of migraine sufferers have depression and about 50 percent have anxiety, although experts are still unsure why this is. Theories propose that hormones or brain chemicals such as serotonin may play a part. Serotonin is a neurotransmitter—it helps the brain cells send messages. One theory about migraines is that the brain releases abnormal amounts of serotonin. Theories about mental illness propose that an imbalance in serotonin is also a factor in depression and anxiety, so serotonin could be contributing to depression, anxiety, and migraines all at the same time.

In support of these theories, doctors also know that some medicines used to treat depression can be effective in treating migraines, although many patients need one medication for their mental illness and another for their migraines. Many doctors also recommend behavioral therapy instead of or in addition to medication to treat anxiety and depression. Further research is needed to determine the nature of the link between migraines and mental illness.

A High Price Tag

Another burden on migraine patients is the cost of caring for this condition. Health insurance covers many of these costs, but not all. For some people, even though evaluation, treatment, and medicines are available, they cannot afford the expense that could provide relief from migraines.

Some insurance plans limit the number of pills a person can receive each month. This leads some

Generic versus Name Brand

Pharmaceutical companies spend a great deal of time and money on drug research. When a new drug is discovered, the company applies for a U.S. patent. A patent identifies the company as the owner and inventor of that drug. It also prevents other companies from producing that drug for 20 years. An example is a prescription drug called Imitrex, which is used to treat migraines. When a new prescription drug becomes available in pharmacies, it is generally expensive at first. Pharmaceutical companies say they price a new drug to pay for the research that discovered and tested it. The price also includes advertising and information needed to launch the new drug. However, many experts have criticized drug companies for overpricing their products.

After a few years, the price of a drug generally goes down slightly. When a drug's patent expires after 20 years, other companies may begin manufacturing and selling that drug. These companies may not use the same brand name as the company that invented it. Instead, they must use the chemical name of the drug. In the case of Imitrex, the chemical name is sumatriptan.

When a drug is sold by another company under the chemical name, it is called a generic drug. It must have the same chemical formula and properties as the original drug. When more companies begin selling the same drug, the price generally comes down due to competition for sales. The result is a savings to the consumer.

people to make hard decisions about whether to take the medication. They fear that if a headache is not a migraine, they have wasted a pill. Some of these people wait to take a pill until they are certain they are getting a migraine, but this delay can make the medication less effective or not work at all. Migraine medications can cost anywhere from $14 to $1,200, depending on whether a person is using pills, nasal spray, or injections. Many people have asked their doctor to prescribe a less expensive drug, even if what they were given was effective. Some people get several migraines per month, so the costs multiply quickly. Those costs are simply too high for some people. Because some migraine medications are very new, less expensive generic drugs are not always available.

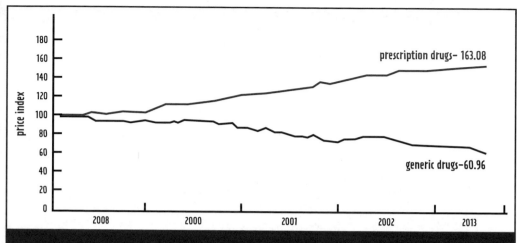

This information from *Mother Jones* shows the difference in price index, or average price, for generic and prescription drugs (in dollars).

On Migraine.com, an author using the name The Migraine Girl wrote about her experience with the high price of her migraine medication. Because her migraines made her throw up, she could not take pills; she would throw them up before they could be effectively absorbed into her body. Her doctor prescribed her a nasal spray called Zomig that worked well. One day when she had run out of Zomig and was experiencing a migraine, her father went to the pharmacy to pick up some more for her. He called her to let her know it would be $171—much more than the $10 she had paid for it previously. This is because in the past, she had already met her deductible, which is an amount of money insurance companies require a person to pay before they will start covering certain costs. For instance, if The Migraine Girl's deductible was $500, she would have to spend that amount of money on health costs before her insurance would cover any medication, surgery, doctor's appointments, or other health costs. The deductible varies from plan to plan; generally the lower the deductible, the higher the monthly fee, which is called a premium.

Deductibles reset every year, so even if someone has met their deductible in the past, they may not meet it in the future, which causes uncertainty for patients about the yearly costs of their health care. Because The Migraine Girl had not met her deductible for that year, her insurance would not fully cover her Zomig; it would cover only half, and she would have to pay the other half—$171. She could not afford to spend that amount on her medication at that time, so her father bought it for her. However, not everyone has a relative who can afford to do this for them.

Research indicates that taking migraine medication in a timely manner can actually save money in the long run. When a person can take medication and avoid a migraine, they are less likely to lose time at work and other activities. In addition, blocking a migraine may reduce the need to visit an emergency room in the event of an extreme headache. However, the up-front cost is sometimes too much for someone to pay, which is why many people have called for insurance companies to change their coverage policies.

When Kids Get Migraines

The symptoms and severity of migraines can be frightening for adults, but they can be even more upsetting for children and teens. About 10 percent of children under age 15 experience migraines, but when a migraine hits, especially for the first time, children are often scared by the extreme pain and might worry about what is happening. They might fear they are going to die and are likely to wonder why such a painful headache is happening to them.

Children and young adults may wish to talk with teachers, coaches, or a school nurse about their migraines or have a parent or guardian do it for them. They might explain that the headaches are real, not just an excuse to get out of school.

Parents can give instructions about how to help the child when a migraine hits, such as ensuring that any medication is taken quickly or allowing the child to lie down or take other measures. A note or instructions from the child's doctor is generally helpful in explaining the situation to teachers or other adults.

Children and teens should be actively involved in managing their migraines. The more young people understand about migraines, the more they can help prevent their attacks. They can watch for and avoid food and environmental triggers. This also helps the child or teen feel more in control of their headaches and feel less victimized by them. Young people can be taught to recognize the warning signs of a

When Medication Causes Headaches

Some people experience an unwelcome side effect of taking medication. Those who take pain medication more than two or three times a week to treat migraines sometimes suffer from a rebound headache. Doctors refer to these as medication-overuse headaches or rebound headaches because the medication seems to bounce back at the patient and cause, rather than cure, a headache. According to the Mayo Clinic, this problem is unique to head pain:

> It appears that any medication taken for pain relief can cause rebound headaches, but only if you already have a headache disorder. Pain relievers taken regularly for another condition, such as arthritis, have not been shown to cause rebound headaches in people who never had a headache disorder.[1]

Rebound headaches are not the same as drug addiction, in which the body craves a certain medication. Rebound headaches sometimes include nausea, irritability, anxiety, or restlessness. A person who suspects they are experiencing this should contact their doctor and likely will need to stop taking the medication; generally, as soon as this happens, the rebound headaches go away. A doctor can work with a patient to find a better pain management solution.

1. Mayo Clinic Staff, "Rebound Headaches," Mayo Clinic, December 2, 2014. www.mayoclinic.org/diseases-conditions/rebound-headaches/basics/definition/con-20024096.

migraine and should thoroughly understand how to respond by taking medication or other steps to block the migraine.

Finding the Right Treatment

Because every person is unique, no medication can cure every migraine every time. Migraine patients typically go through a trial-and-error period with their doctors. A doctor will suggest medication based on the patient's symptoms and health history. The patient can then use that medication and judge its effectiveness. Some patients get lucky and have success right away. Others may find no relief at all, even after trying several drugs.

Communication with a doctor is important. When a medication is unsuccessful, the doctor should be notified so a different medication can be prescribed. The doctor should also be contacted if the medication produces unpleasant side effects, such as drowsiness, aches, inability to sleep, or jitteriness. Some patients are willing to live with mild side effects if the medication is highly effective. Other side effects may be unbearable and require a medication to be stopped.

Finding a helpful migraine medication requires patience. It may require sampling a number of different drugs to find one that works. A migraine journal can be useful in this process. By recording any changes in migraines along with any side effects, the patient and doctor can evaluate medications and find the best solution.

CHAPTER FOUR

TREATING MIGRAINES

Today, many medications are available to diagnose and treat migraines, but this is a relatively recent development. People knew their head hurt but did not always know why, although they may still have been able to identify migraine triggers before there was a term for such things. They tried many things that were often untested by science to treat their migraines. For example, an ancient Egyptian headache remedy was to place a clay model of a crocodile atop the patient's head. The crocodile's mouth was filled with grain, and then a strip of linen bearing the names of the gods was wrapped under the patient's chin and over the head to tie the crocodile in place. Researchers today believe that if this worked, it may have been due to the pressure of the figurine and the cooling effect of the clay.

Other home, or folk, remedies consisted of treatments that patients could make in their own kitchens with local ingredients. Some folk remedies for migraines include inhaling vinegar fumes; massaging menthol, eucalyptus oil, peppermint oil, or rosemary oil on the forehead; or consuming a tea made from cayenne pepper, celery seeds, or ginger. Soaking a person's feet in hot water containing powdered mustard is another remedy, as is eating a few teaspoons of honey at each meal. Some of these treatments are still recommended for people who prefer not to take medicine, although they have not been scientifically tested and estimating their success is difficult. In recent times, some doctors have begun to look to folk remedies and judge whether they might have merit. They realize that in many cases, folk remedies were actually effective and could be studied for current uses. For instance, people used to chew on willow bark to cure their headaches. In 1829, it was discovered that this is because the bark contains an ingredient called salicin, which has pain-relieving properties similar to aspirin. As science advanced, it became possible to extract the salicin from the bark and make medication.

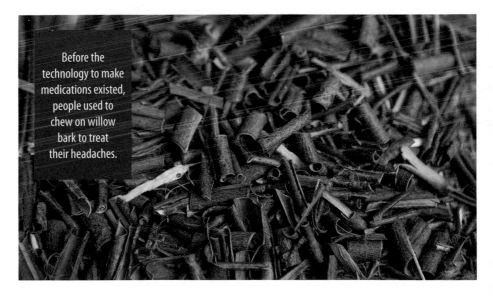

Before the technology to make medications existed, people used to chew on willow bark to treat their headaches.

With so many people suffering from migraines, cures are highly sought after. Numerous treatments have been suggested, and some of them date back hundreds of years. No treatment should be attempted without the supervision of a doctor or a trusted adult. Some treatments are appropriate for certain people but could be dangerous for others. A person's size, weight, age, allergies, and other medical conditions, such as asthma or heart disease, are all considered when a doctor recommends treatment.

Multiple Approaches to Migraine Management

According to experts, there are two main aspects to migraine management: treatment and prevention. Because no single cure exists for every migraine and because every person has different experiences, multiple approaches offer the best chance of preventing, blocking, and treating migraines.

Preventive treatments might involve a number of strategies, such as maintaining healthy blood pressure, exercising, and eating a healthy diet. Prevention can also include taking regular medications to stop migraines before they start. When migraines are prevented from taking hold, patients experience the least amount of pain and the best quality of life. Researchers are always looking for new methods to prevent migraines and allow patients to avoid the headaches altogether.

Trigger management involves helping migraine patients identify some or all of the triggers that set off a migraine. Recognizing foods or activities that start a migraine and then avoiding them can be highly effective for some patients.

In the past several decades, a number of new medications have been developed that can block a migraine before it fully takes hold. These prescription drugs are known as abortive treatments. Generally in the form of pills or nasal sprays, these treatments are taken as soon as the patient recognizes the signs of a migraine. The success rates of minimizing or completely canceling a headache are very good. These treatments are most successful when taken promptly after warning signs begin. When patients wait longer, the effectiveness of the medicines is not as high.

General pain management is needed when a migraine begins and progresses out of control. Even with preventive treatment, people are sometimes

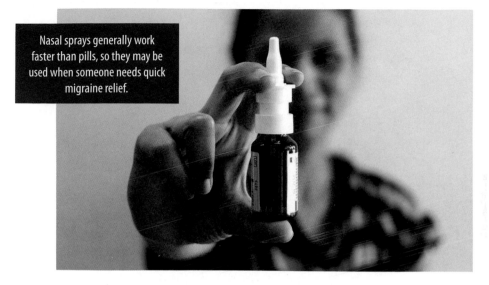

Nasal sprays generally work faster than pills, so they may be used when someone needs quick migraine relief.

unable to avoid migraines, and some people must endure them while they figure out which treatment and prevention methods work for them. Many treatments are available to lessen migraine pain, including over-the-counter medicines, prescription drugs, and other therapies.

Lifestyle Changes

Many possible treatments exist for migraines. Because migraines are so individualized, certain treatments work for some people but not for others. The best results come when a doctor and patient work together and test the various treatments. Treatments that offer no relief can be discarded, and those that lessen migraines can be followed more seriously. Most patients will test a variety of methods, ignore those that are not helpful, and incorporate those that lessen the pain or frequency of migraines. Several medicines currently exist for treating migraines. Some of these can be purchased in a drugstore or grocery store. Others require a prescription from a doctor. All medications carry certain risks, so children under age 18 should never take medicines without the permission of a parent, doctor, or trusted adult. Selecting a medication can be tricky and depends on a person's other health factors.

Many people prefer to start with non-drug preventive treatments first and only add medication if it is absolutely necessary. Additionally, some people's migraines are resistant to medication; according to *Prevention* magazine, "Even the best medication we have doesn't work for one-third of sufferers."[18] Using non-drug methods can also help people take their medication less frequently, which can prevent rebound headaches. Whether alone or in combination with medicine, there are several lifestyle changes people can make to potentially improve their migraines.

Diet is one important aspect of migraine management as well as overall health. Every day, Americans hear messages that a healthy diet is important for the human body to function properly. Eating fruits and vegetables, avoiding junk food, and maintaining a proper weight all help regulate blood pressure, boost the immune system, and provide energy. These steps can help a person to avoid problems such as heart disease, stroke, and diabetes. A migraine patient who follows a healthy diet improves their chances of successfully avoiding migraines. This includes eliminating any trigger foods from the diet.

Skipping meals is generally considered to be unhealthy, and it can sometimes bring on a migraine. This is a problem that can generally be avoided. Some patients keep healthy snacks handy in case they miss a meal. When a meal is unavoidably missed, patients typically take steps to eat as soon as possible or perhaps take medication to block a possible migraine.

The human body needs a number of specific vitamins and minerals in order to function and be healthy. Most of these are found in foods, but processed foods and fast foods tend to lose vitamins and minerals. Many migraine patients consult with a doctor to learn about vitamins or minerals. A doctor may recommend a multivitamin once per day or may advise other specific combinations of vitamins or minerals. Magnesium is considered especially important for people suffering from migraines, and it is found in nuts; beans; dark green, leafy vegetables; and whole-grain foods.

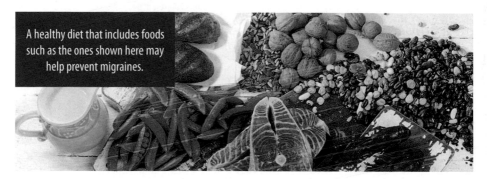

A healthy diet that includes foods such as the ones shown here may help prevent migraines.

Vitamin B2, also known as riboflavin, is also highly recommended by experts. Studies have shown that getting about 400 milligrams of B2 per day can be effective in preventing migraines. Other vitamins and supplements that have been studied include vitamin D, which may play a role in the way people feel pain; butterbur, an herb that can help prevent migraine attacks if 75 milligrams are taken twice a day; feverfew, which helps reduce migraine pain; and ginger, which helps reduce nausea. Feverfew and ginger have been combined into a tablet called LipiGesic, which has been found in one study to shorten the duration of a migraine attack.

Along with a healthy diet, doctors have known for many years that water is essential to good health. The human body is about 60 percent water, and the brain is about 75 percent water. Water inside the body helps in healing, eliminating wastes, and delivering nutrients to the cells. When a person does not drink enough water, dehydration sets in. This can cause stomachache, muscle cramps, headache, and dizziness. Migraine sufferers are wise to stay hydrated as a step to avoid headaches. A properly hydrated brain may be less likely to experience disturbances in the levels of brain chemicals.

Taking Care of the Body

Doctors recommend exercise for nearly everyone. Walking, bike riding, swimming, and playing sports help keep the heart and muscles healthy. For people with migraines, regular exercise can help by keeping the body in shape, regulating blood sugar, and maintaining energy.

In some patients, however, exercise can set off a migraine. Strenuous exercise, such as weight lifting, running a marathon, or pushups, could start a headache. This is more common in men than women. For these patients, a migraine journal can be an important tool. By recording the types and levels of exercise and comparing them to the migraine onset, patterns can be discovered. A patient can then design an exercise plan to maintain health while avoiding migraines.

Sleep is also important, but most American adults and teens do not get the amount of sleep recommended by doctors. Researchers are beginning to identify and understand the problems associated with a lack of sleep. Some people prone to migraines have discovered that too much or too little sleep can start a migraine. In order to prevent migraines, a person needs to understand their personal sleep requirements. Recording sleep habits in a migraine journal can help identify this relationship. When a migraine occurs, the journal can be consulted to determine whether the person has been in a pattern of too much or too little sleep. The person can then take steps to regulate sleeping habits and attempt to avoid migraines.

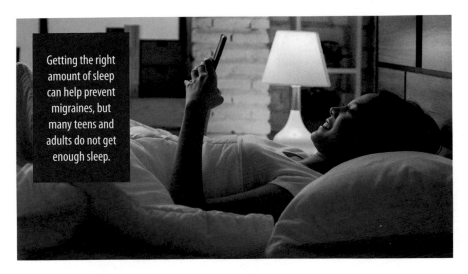

Getting the right amount of sleep can help prevent migraines, but many teens and adults do not get enough sleep.

Alternative Treatments

Some treatments have been around for thousands of years and, for many people, are effective in reducing stress, which is a known migraine trigger. Everyone manages stress differently depending on their personality. Some people seek ways to reduce stress by staying organized, keeping lists, asking others for help, and managing the number of events in their schedules. They might also find ways to unwind from stress, such as taking a bath, listening to music, spending time with friends or family, or setting aside personal time each day.

Meditation is one alternative treatment that is recommended for many ailments—not only migraines, but depression, anxiety, and general stress. Meditation involves slowing down the breath and focusing on one thing, such as breathing pattern or a repeated word or phrase called a mantra. When meditation is done successfully, this focus and slow breathing combine to block out distractions and reduce stress. However, meditation does not work for everyone; some people find that a better way to relax and reduce their stress is to distract themselves with something they enjoy, such as a movie, book, or puzzle. Adult coloring books have become increasingly popular in recent years for this reason: They allow someone to sit quietly while still focusing on something outside themselves. For many people, coloring becomes a form of meditation.

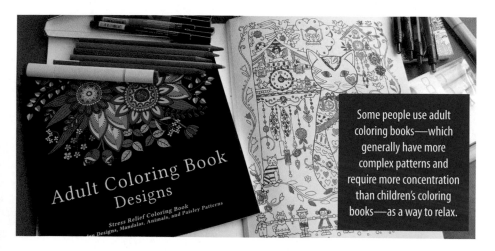

Some people use adult coloring books—which generally have more complex patterns and require more concentration than children's coloring books—as a way to relax.

Similarly, yoga and tai chi are often recommended as ways to reduce stress. Yoga is an ancient system of exercise that originated in India and incorporates breathing and meditation. It involves moving the body into various poses. The body benefits from stretching and gaining flexibility. Muscles are also exercised while holding a yoga pose; when a participant works to maintain balance in the pose, the muscles must work to hold the body in place. Yoga is considered a low-impact workout because it does not stress the joints.

Tai chi is a martial art from China. It also places emphasis on breathing, balance, and meditation. It is low impact and easy on joints, such as knees and elbows. Tai chi also offers flexibility and stretching. Both of these exercises can be beneficial to migraine sufferers. Because they are gentle exercise, they avoid bringing on headaches the way strenuous exercise, such as running or weight lifting, can. Some patients report that yoga or tai chi helps them relax from stress and thus reduces the chance of getting a migraine. However, like meditation, these practices are not for everyone. People must experiment to find what works for them personally.

Tension in the muscles, particularly in the head and neck, is believed to bring on migraines for some people. Relaxation techniques can help people learn to release tension when they are under stress and thus avoid migraines. Massage is also known to relieve muscle tension. Some people seek out a full massage from a professional, but others learn simple techniques they can practice on themselves, such as massaging the head and neck.

People with weak muscles, with physical abnormalities, or who have experienced migraines following an accident may find relief with physical therapy. A licensed physical therapist can help strengthen, stretch, or relax muscles, especially in the neck and shoulders. Physical therapists are trained to analyze the way muscles move and identify problems with strength, posture, and symmetry. They can teach a patient exercises that will correct any number of problems with the muscles or skeleton. Correcting certain physical problems can sometimes help relieve migraines.

Practiced for centuries in China, acupuncture is a technique in which tiny needles—some only as thick as a human hair—are inserted into the skin at key locations. The process is said to free the passage of energy—known as chi—that flows through the body. Many people say they have experienced relief from acupuncture for conditions such as arthritis, back pain, menstrual cramps, and migraines.

Migraine patient Miya Kressin has had favorable results in relieving her migraines after acupuncture. Hoping to get some relief from fluid retention, she visited an acupuncturist. After several visits she noticed that her migraines were not coming as often. Kressin said,

> *I told my acupuncturist that my migraines had gotten better. He said, "Why didn't you tell me you had migraines?" He adjusted my treatments and I could see immediate results. Now, when I feel a migraine coming on, I get to him as quickly as possible. By inserting only three needles in my forehead, he can either block a migraine entirely or reduce the pain level.*[19]

According to Dr. Hansa Bhargava, studies have "found some evidence that acupuncture may relieve pain during an acute migraine episode and may modestly reduce frequency."[20] As with all other treatments, individual results tend to vary.

Avoiding Scams

When looking for treatments, especially those that are less common, migraine patients must be careful to do their research before spending money. Unfortunately, some people see an opportunity to take advantage of migraine sufferers who are looking for relief, and they may try to sell products that either do not work or are actually harmful in some cases. One example is an email advertisement for a booklet called *The Migraine Protocol*, "supposedly authored by a Jenny Appleton, a migraine sufferer with apparently no credentials other than that she's had

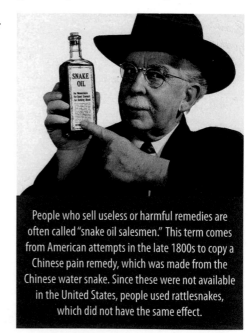

People who sell useless or harmful remedies are often called "snake oil salesmen." This term comes from American attempts in the late 1800s to copy a Chinese pain remedy, which was made from the Chinese water snake. Since these were not available in the United States, people used rattlesnakes, which did not have the same effect.

crippling migraines since age 16."[21] The advertisement offers the booklet, which claims to be able to
guarantee the complete elimination of the customer's migraines, for $39. Several things are common to
scams such as this:

- They include promises of miraculous, guaranteed
  cures for little or no effort.
- It is difficult or impossible to find information
  online about the author or company selling
  the product.
- Reviews for the product are overwhelmingly positive or negative. Some review websites are set up
  specifically to give good reviews of the product,
  and these will all have five-star reviews with links
  to the product's website. On reputable websites,
  all or most of the reviews will have one-star rat-
  ings describing how the product did not work
  as advertised.
- They claim "Big Pharma [a negative nickname
  for pharmaceutical companies] doesn't want
  you to know about it and no medical journal or
  expert will put their name on the product out of
  fear that 'Pharma Bullies' will retaliate."[22] This is
  done to explain to the customer why they have
  never heard of the product before and why no
  recommendations from experts can be found.
  Additionally, setting up a product as controver-
  sial or secret often makes people more interested
  in it, especially since many people already distrust
  pharmaceutical companies.
- The product is being sold for an amount of money
  that is higher than average. For instance, $39 may
  not seem like much, but since information about
  migraines can be found for free on various reputable medical websites or in medical books that
  can be borrowed from a library, the cost is much
  more than the product is worth.

Michael Shames, the founder of San Diego Consumers' Action Network, noted that consumers should "beware ANY Net-based sales pitch that has uncredentialed, slick video presentations with no independent reviews. It may not be a scam, but it is probably a rip-off because it is overpriced for what it is offering."[23]

Finding Emotional Support

People who experience migraines deal not only with pain but also with the guilt and frustration of missing activities or work because of their headaches. Some places offer support groups for migraine sufferers. These groups help people deal with their feelings by sharing their stories, advice, and worries with others in the same situation.

Local migraine support groups can often be found by searching something such as "migraine support groups in Chicago" or "migraine support groups near [zip code]." If someone lives in an area where there are none close by, they may choose to start one themselves or participate in an online support group. These are generally set up as forums where anyone can make posts and reply to others. Always ask a parent or guardian before participating in an online forum or joining a support group.

Common Migraine Medications

Aspirin, ibuprofen, and acetaminophen are three common OTC pain relievers. For some people with migraines, these can be taken when the headache is just starting so it does not get worse. Described by doctors as "the wonder drug," aspirin can relieve pain and swelling. It is also a blood thinner, which means it reduces the blood's ability to clot. Aspirin is sometimes recommended to prevent strokes or heart attacks. Some migraine sufferers take aspirin to relieve pain; they sometimes combine it with caffeine.

Because it is a blood thinner, aspirin must be avoided by anyone who has had recent surgery or has a clotting disorder. It should not be taken by children or teens who have recently had viral illnesses, such as chicken pox or the flu, due to the risk of developing Reye's syndrome. This potentially fatal complication is a rare disorder that causes brain and liver damage. It is most often seen in children who take aspirin during or immediately after having a viral infection. When taken safely in the absence of these situations, some people prone to migraines find relief from aspirin.

Commonly known by the brand name Tylenol, acetaminophen is a popular medicine for relieving pain and lowering fever. Acetaminophen is available in liquid form for infants, chewable tablets for children, and higher-strength pills for teens and adults. Acetaminophen reduces headache pain in some migraine sufferers. It is available in drugstores, grocery stores, and discount stores without a prescription. It is combined with stronger medications in the prescription pain relievers Vicodin and Percocet. Acetaminophen is generally considered to be safe in the correct doses. Patients who consume extremely high doses of acetaminophen or who take it while drinking alcohol run the risk of liver damage, which can be fatal.

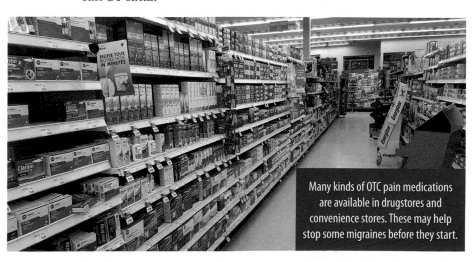

Many kinds of OTC pain medications are available in drugstores and convenience stores. These may help stop some migraines before they start.

Sold under the brand names Advil and Motrin, ibuprofen is a popular remedy for headaches, body aches, and fevers. Like aspirin, ibuprofen is favored for its ability to reduce swelling. Many migraine sufferers use ibuprofen to treat their headaches. "If I can take enough ibuprofen quickly, as soon as I recognize a migraine, I can usually reduce the headache to a point that I can function,"[24] said Deborah Weaver, who suffers from migraines. Other people with moderate migraines report similar success when ibuprofen is taken early. Current research shows that for some people, ibuprofen is more effective when taken with caffeine.

Other effective medications work in similar ways but require a prescription. Nonsteroidal anti-inflammatory drugs (NSAIDs) are often prescribed for migraine; these reduce pain and inflammation—swelling and redness caused by injury, which can make pain worse. Aspirin and ibuprofen are NSAIDs; acetaminophen only treats pain, not inflammation. Prescription-strength NSAIDs are often prescribed to treat more severe migraines.

Some medications are prescribed to treat other symptoms of migraine, such as nausea and dizziness. For instance, if someone has difficulty keeping food or pills down when they have a migraine, they may be prescribed an antinausea medication such as ondansetron, a pill that works quickly to calm nausea so pain medication can be taken effectively. Others get around this by using nasal sprays. In addition, nasal sprays generally work faster than pills because they are absorbed into the body more quickly. People who have severe migraine pain and need immediate relief may choose nasal sprays for this reason. When Terrell Davis got a migraine during Super Bowl XXXII, he used a nasal spray that allowed him to get back in the game.

The Opioid Problem

Some migraine sufferers who have moderate to severe pain and do not respond to the most common medications may be prescribed opioids. This is a class of painkiller that comes from the opium poppy, such as morphine. Opioids are very strong and highly addictive; in recent years, it has become clear that overprescription of opioids for less severe pain has resulted in an addiction epidemic. Although the majority of people who are prescribed opioids use them responsibly, between 8 and 12 percent become addicted, according to the National Institute on Drug Abuse (NIDA). This can lead to the use of heroin, which is cheaper and more widely available than prescription opioids. To address this, doctors are trying to prescribe them less often, but some people need them to function in daily life. The National Headache Foundation offers guidelines for the responsible use of opioids:

- *Take the medication only as directed by a medical doctor or other qualified healthcare professional*

- *Evaluate the benefits and risks of each medication with a healthcare provider before it is prescribed*

- *Do not increase the recommended dose or frequency of opioids*

- *Do not take opioids for a longer time than a healthcare provider has directed*

- *Consult with a healthcare provider before abruptly ending opioid use*[1]

1. "Responsible Use of Opioids," National Headache Foundation, November 19, 2007. www.headaches.org/2007/11/19/responsible-use-of-opioids/.

Other Types of Medication

A category of drug known as triptans is designed to control the behavior of serotonin. Triptans are available in about eight different forms. The most commonly used form is called frovatriptan (Frova); according to 2017 guidelines from the US Headache Consortium, a group made up of experts from the American Academy of Neurology and the American Headache Society, it is one of the first medications that should be recommended for migraines. Other commonly prescribed triptans include sumatriptan (Imitrex) and zolmitriptan (Zomig). Triptans are effective in relieving headaches, photophobia, phonophobia, and nausea, and they help enable patients to engage in normal activities. They "are considered selective serotonin receptor agonists, meaning that triptans work by stimulating serotonin … to reduce inflammation and constrict blood vessels, thereby stopping the headache or migraine."[25]

While triptans are known to be effective for many people, some trial and error in the timing is required for patients who get auras. Researchers are still unsure whether they are most effective if taken before, during, or after aura symptoms begin, so it may take a few tries for someone to get the best effect. Additionally, triptans are not safe when used to treat brain stem or hemiplegic migraines; this is why the term "complex migraine," which included multiple kinds of migraine with aura, is no longer preferred. Getting an exact diagnosis is important when determining what kind of medication is best to use. Triptans continue to be researched, and new forms are being developed and tested. They may cause mild side effects, including numbness, dizziness, dry mouth, and sleepiness.

When a single medicine fails to have an effect on migraines, some doctors turn to combination medicines. Aspirin and acetaminophen, for example, can be purchased in combination without a prescription, sometimes with caffeine added. This product is sometimes labeled specifically as a migraine medication.

With a doctor's prescription, acetaminophen and other drugs are available combined with codeine and other pain relievers. Some well-known names are Vicodin and Percocet. Numerous combination medications are available by prescription. Before prescribing them for a patient, a doctor must consider the patient's other health issues. These medications have the potential to become addictive, so doctors and patients must watch for signs of dependency and take steps to prevent addiction.

Off-Label Medications

When a medication is prescribed to treat something other than what it is marketed for, it is called prescribing off-label. Some medications that were created to treat one ailment have side effects that can treat a different one as well. For instance, two types of medications intended to treat high blood pressure, or hypertension, have been successful in treating migraines. One of these is called a beta blocker and is available under various brand names, including Sectral, Tenormin, Lopressor, and Blocadren. Beta blockers help regulate the heartbeat and dilate the blood vessels. They have a variety of minor side effects, including weakness, dizziness, diarrhea or constipation, sleepiness, cold hands and feet, and upset stomach.

The other hypertension medication that is effective for migraines is called a calcium channel blocker. It also comes in different forms under several brand names. Calcium channel blockers work to block serotonin, which prevents blood vessels from constricting. Calcium channel blockers are generally only prescribed after other medications have been tried because some people's migraines increase when they first start using this medicine. Doctors and patients need to work together closely to judge the effectiveness of the medication and discuss any side effects as well as monitor blood pressure and heart health.

A recent development in the treatment of migraines is the use of neurotoxins. A neurotoxin is a substance that causes damage to the nerves or tissues. In the case of migraines, a neurotoxin known by the brand name Botox is used. Botox comes from the botulinum toxin, which causes a type of food poisoning called botulism. Botulism can be fatal, but Botox is not dangerous because the poison is injected into the skin, not digested in the stomach.

When Botox is injected into the body, it weakens or paralyzes muscles. It is most commonly known as a treatment for facial wrinkles—wrinkles are less noticeable when certain muscles in the face are paralyzed. Botox has also been used to treat medical conditions. The use of Botox for migraines was discovered accidentally when people who received Botox injections reported that their migraine symptoms were lessened. However, it only works for people who get chronic migraines. People who experience headaches fewer than 15 days per month or who more often get other kinds of headaches, such as cluster headaches, will not benefit from this treatment.

For treatment of migraines, Botox is injected into the muscles above the brow, across the forehead, around the eyes, on the sides of the head, and on the back of the head near the neck. Doctors are still studying this procedure to determine the most effective injection sites. Botox injections last for three to four months and then must be repeated. Each treatment may involve as many as 40 injections. Researchers are trying to understand the link between this treatment and the success in relieving migraines; the current theory is that by paralyzing the muscles, Botox stops nerve cells from transmitting pain messages.

Although antidepressants are intended to relieve depression and prevent mood swings, several are also prescribed to prevent migraines. The different types of antidepressants that are available affect different mechanisms inside the brain. Some of these mechanisms regulate serotonin. Tricyclic antidepressants are currently considered to be the most effective at preventing migraines. However, despite their success with migraine relief, some of these medications have a number of side effects. Some of these are mild, including dry mouth, drowsiness, and increased appetite, but the most serious possible side effect is an increase in suicidal thoughts. The use of antidepressants must be considered carefully in migraine patients. The link between migraines and depression is currently an area of high interest for further study.

Some migraine patients have found relief from their headaches by taking antiseizure medicines. A seizure is a disturbance in the brain's natural electric field that causes abnormal behavior. Seizures can range from short blackouts to episodes of uncontrolled kicking and thrashing, and they can be dangerous. Seizures can be caused by several different conditions, including a disorder called epilepsy, which brings on frequent seizures. Migraines are not considered to be related to seizures, but certain antiseizure medications have been found to reduce the number of migraines a person has. These medications help prevent neurotransmitters in the brain from overfiring. They are taken daily as a preventative medication, but the dosage of each pill must be small to prevent side effects such as nausea, shaking, weight gain, hair loss, and memory problems.

Unproven Treatments

Some treatments are less common and are rumored to work but have not been scientifically proven. Some people say they have been successful at treating their migraines with these methods, while others say they have had no result.

One such treatment is called biofeedback, which is the theory that humans can be taught to control involuntary body mechanisms. This practice requires professional training and demands time and patience. To learn biofeedback, a person is fitted with sensors that monitor heart rate, breathing, and blood pressure. By engaging in several relaxation techniques, a person can learn to regulate blood pressure, skin temperature, and heart rate. In addition to providing relaxation, biofeedback can sometimes be used to slow or block the early stages of a migraine. This technique requires months or years to learn and is not a quick fix for migraines. Not all patients who attempt to learn biofeedback are successful.

Another treatment that promotes relaxation is aromatherapy, which is the use of scented essential oils. Some people claim that smelling certain scents, such as lavender or peppermint oil, can reduce pain. While aromatherapy has few negative side effects, many say there is also little evidence of essential oils having a direct effect on pain. However, a person may benefit from aromatherapy if certain scents relax them, and that relaxation contributes to fewer migraines.

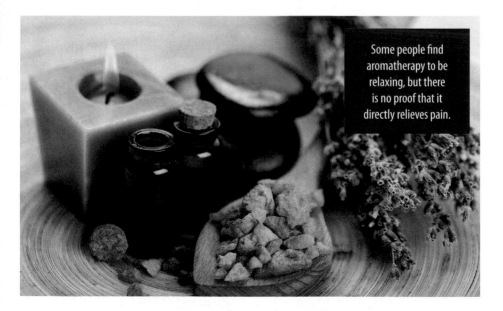

Some people find aromatherapy to be relaxing, but there is no proof that it directly relieves pain.

A third treatment with uncertain effectiveness is a daith piercing. The daith is part of the stiff cartilage near the middle of a person's ear, and it is rumored to

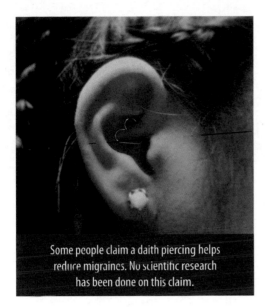

Some people claim a daith piercing helps reduce migraines. No scientific research has been done on this claim.

contain a pressure point that relieves migraines when it is pierced. Some people have said it has worked, while others say it has not or are unsure. If people want a daith piercing for aesthetic reasons, there is nothing wrong with getting one, but experts do not recommend that someone get one specifically to try treating their migraines.

Migraines are like an enormous puzzle. Their wide range of different symptoms must first be analyzed to see the picture of a migraine. Then, by experimenting with various lifestyle techniques and medications, a doctor and patient can start to sort the pieces into a reasonable order. Sometimes, pieces have to be thrown away entirely or pieces are missing. Patience and persistence are two of the most important tools when trying to understand migraines and prevent their return.

CHAPTER FIVE

CONTINUING RESEARCH

Although many people around the world experience migraines, the condition is still not well understood. It can be difficult for patients to find accurate information online, which means they may end up trying ineffective or dangerous treatments on their own rather than consulting a doctor. Additionally, myths about migraines and people who suffer from them persist because so little information is publicly available.

Joel Saper, a neurologist with the Michigan Headache and Neurological Institute in Ann Arbor, has encountered this problem. He expressed his gratitude to the Migraine Research Foundation, which was founded in 2007, for its role in encouraging and funding migraine research. According to Saper,

> Migraine is under-researched by the scientific community, under-treated by physicians, and under-appreciated by society. There is no condition of such magnitude, yet so shrouded in myth, misinformation, and mistreatment, as migraine. The Migraine Research Foundation is about more than just the research that it will fund directly—it is about stimulating others to join us in addressing a critical gap in medical research.[26]

By continuing to research migraines, experts may find new ways to diagnose and treat them. Research might focus on the causes, triggers, or process of migraines; the prevention of migraines; or ways to halt migraines that have already begun. The field of migraine research is extremely broad, but any area of research could provide a breakthrough at any time.

Studying the Brain

Modern testing that allows doctors to see inside the body is critical to migraine research. MRIs, CT scans, and even X-rays allow researchers to learn more about what a migraine is and what it is not. Newer tests that may impact migraine research are also in development.

The single-photon emission computerized tomography (SPECT) scan is a modern test that lets doctors watch the function of internal organs. In this test, a patient consumes a radioactive substance; as that substance travels through the body, doctors can scan and record the behavior of organs.

Observation of the brain during a SPECT scan can help diagnose Alzheimer's disease, strokes, and seizures. SPECT scans are especially good at mapping the blood supply inside the brain; the radioactive material remains in the blood and does not enter the tissues in the brain. A SPECT scan can help diagnose migraines by ruling out other possible conditions. SPECT scans may also help future research.

Ongoing Research

Finding an effective treatment for any disease takes time. Even when new treatments are proposed, they must be studied and tested. Test subjects must be located with the correct sets of symptoms, and they must be healthy enough to attempt a new treatment. Patients who undergo new treatments must be monitored to gauge the success of the treatment, watched for any side effects, and followed to learn of any long-term effects. For a treatment to become recognized and accepted, it also needs to gain the approval of the U.S. Food and Drug Administration (FDA).

The procedure known as occipital nerve stimulation was first used in 1977, but it is still considered a developing treatment for chronic migraines. In this procedure, a surgeon implants a small device at the base of the skull, near the occipital nerve. Special wires are threaded under the skin to connect this device to a pulse generator; this is also implanted under the skin, generally under the collarbone, at the lower back, or in the lower abdomen. The pulse generator sends electrical impulses to the occipital nerve. These pulses might be sent in a steady stream or only as needed.

Occipital nerve stimulation has improved headaches for some people who have tried it, but the results have not been consistent. Additionally, tests have been done only in very small numbers, and long-term results are not available. Occipital nerve stimulation requires surgery and comes with a risk of infection. In some cases, the implanted wires must be replaced or adjusted. More studies are needed before this procedure can become a common treatment.

Another treatment that is being studied is transcranial magnetic stimulation (TMS). Researchers have found that administering magnetic pulses to migraine sufferers appeared to stop the wave of neuron excitation that is believed to lead off a migraine. Not many studies have been done on it yet, but in one study of "267 people who had migraine with aura, more than a third of those who used TMS were pain-free after 2 hours, compared to 22% who did not get TMS."[27]

TMS involves placing a large electromagnet against the patient's head. The magnet sends painless electric currents through the brain. It was first created as a treatment for depression in patients who had no success with medications or other treatments. The outcome of TMS and its effects on both depression and migraines supports the idea that these two conditions are linked. Researchers are currently studying TMS as a treatment for a number of brain disorders.

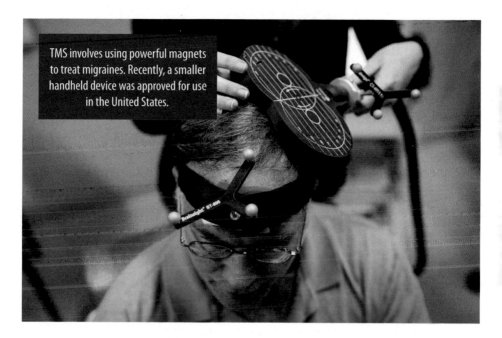

TMS involves using powerful magnets to treat migraines. Recently, a smaller handheld device was approved for use in the United States.

Traditionally, TMS requires a series of half-hour-long treatments several times per week over several weeks or a full month. The effects are believed to be temporary and may last only a few weeks or months. However, in 2013, a company called eNeura made a handheld TMS device called Cerena that people can use at home. A second device by the same company, called SpringTMS, is currently the only one on the U.S. market. WebMD explained,

> To use SpringTMS, you hold both handles on the sides of what looks like a battery-powered box. (A mini version doesn't have handles). You then place the device against the back of your head and push a button. Each magnetic pulse fires a mild electrical current and activates a part of the brain called the "occipital cortex." The treatment is thought to

reduce or halt migraine pain by calming overactive brain activity.[28]

Like all treatments, TMS comes with side effects, including headaches, scalp discomfort, twitchy facial muscles, or lightheadedness. Additionally, it generally only relieves the pain of a migraine, not the other symptoms that go along with it. However, it may provide some relief for people whose migraines are resistant to other treatments.

A Radical Treatment

Just as Botox has been used to treat migraines, some types of plastic surgery have produced positive results in migraine sufferers. This is not a new proposal; in 2009, the medical journal *Plastic and Reconstructive Surgery* issued the results of a study that used plastic surgery as a treatment for migraines. In the study, migraine patients underwent a forehead lift to see if their migraines improved. More than 80 percent of patients found that their migraines occurred less often following surgery. Some had only half as many headaches, and others had fewer or even no headaches at all after the surgery.

This study came about due to the observations of plastic surgeons that their patients reported fewer migraines after forehead lifts. The study offers scientific proof that this type of surgery improves migraines. Neurologists were skeptical at first, but interested. Because migraines are believed to occur deep inside the brain, success with forehead surgery did not make sense. Further research into surgery and Botox led to the theory that migraines are caused by irritation of nerves in the scalp. Since Botox treatments only offer temporary relief, surgery may be an option for people who want something more permanent. A 2014 study showed that using "cosmetic eyelid surgery to

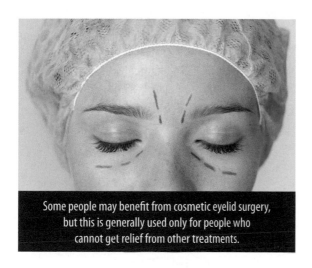

Some people may benefit from cosmetic eyelid surgery, but this is generally used only for people who cannot get relief from other treatments.

decompress, or 'free up' the nerves that trigger migraines … [had a] 90% success rate among patients."[29] Experts say that if people respond to Botox, they are likely to respond to this type of surgery. However, surgery is generally a last resort after other medications have been tried.

Research into this procedure is ongoing. Doctors are excited about the potential of treating migraines through a single surgery, freeing patients from the expense and burden of taking a number of medications. They caution, however, that the surgery is not for everyone and that patients will need to meet certain standards in order to be considered for this technique.

New Medical Breakthroughs

Doctors and researchers never know where or when the next major medical breakthrough will occur. Although new procedures or implants may show promise for migraines, traditional treatments in the form of medications are far from being abandoned. As more is understood about the mechanism of migraines, researchers can target more specific effects inside the brain. Researchers also sometimes revisit older or abandoned therapies to find out whether new information might make older therapies worth a second look.

A medication called dihydroergotamine (DHE) is an approved drug for treating severe migraines.

It is not effective when taken by mouth; it can be given as a nasal spray or injection, but there are issues with these forms as well—for example, administering the medicine intravenously (through an IV) is the fastest and most effective way, but that requires someone to go to a hospital every time they have a migraine. For this reason, researchers are doing trials on a form of DHE with the brand name Levadex that can be inhaled the way asthma medication is.

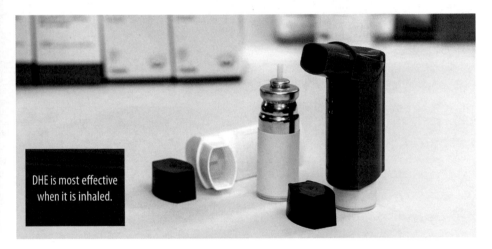

DHE is most effective when it is inhaled.

Another new therapy that shows promise uses antibodies—proteins in the blood that fight bacteria, viruses, and other invaders—to change the way brain chemicals work. One specific chemical, called calcitonin gene-related peptide (CGRP), has been found to play a role in migraine pain as well as sensitivity to light and sound. According to BBC News, "Four drug companies are racing to develop antibodies that neutralise CGRP. Some work by sticking to CGRP, while others block the part of a brain cell with which it interacts."[30] Two antibodies—erenumab and fremanezumab—have shown promise in clinical trials, which are tests on human volunteers. The erenumab trial involved 995 participants, and the fremanezumab trial involved 1,130. BBC News summarized the findings of the trials:

> At the start of the trial the patients had migraines on an average of eight days a month. The [erenumab] study found 50% of those given the antibody injections halved their number of migraine days per month. About 27% did have a similar effect without treatment, which reflects the natural ebb and flow of the disease ...

> [With fremanezumab], 41% of patients halved their number of migraine days compared to 18% without treatment ... The hope is discovering CGRP and precisely targeting it with antibodies should lead to fewer side-effects [than with current treatments]. Both studies say long-term safety data still needs to be studied.[31]

Another therapy that is currently being studied is medical marijuana. Research in this area has been slow because up until recently, marijuana was completely illegal, which made it difficult for researchers to study it. Now that it is legal for medical use in many states, research has progressed, and scientists hope it will eventually be available as a safe, commonly prescribed cure for migraines; however, there is still more to be done. Scientists who have focused on medical marijuana research say that "while using cannabis may not be better than taking conventional prescription medicine for migraine sufferers, the list of side effects is smaller than prescription medication."[32] The active ingredients are tetrahydrocannabinol (THC) and cannabidiol (CBD). THC is the ingredient that creates changes in awareness associated with "getting high," while CBD has been shown to have positive effects on certain physical and mental conditions, such as migraines, epilepsy, and anxiety. For this reason, strains of marijuana are being bred without THC so people can get the medical benefits without getting high. Additionally, concentrated forms of CBD are being developed, such as cannabis oil.

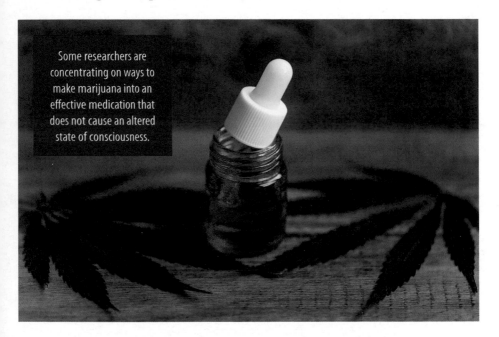

Some researchers are concentrating on ways to make marijuana into an effective medication that does not cause an altered state of consciousness.

Doctors caution people against smoking marijuana to treat their migraines for several reasons, including the legal risk, the high that impairs daily activities, and the fact that dosage varies among plants. According to *Self* magazine, CBD may be sold at some health food stores; however, as with all treatments, this should be discussed with a doctor first.

More to Do

In March 2009, the Migraine Research Foundation announced a new plan to encourage research into migraines in children. The plan, called For Our Children, was designed to provide grant money for pediatric migraine research. It also established a research award for success in pediatric migraine research and a fellowship to encourage new doctors

An Uncertain Connection

Several studies in 2008, 2009, and 2014 showed that women who get migraines have a 30–60 percent lower risk for breast cancer. Researchers cannot explain the connection yet. The 2014 study noted that the link is more specific than was previously thought; women whose migraines start before age 20 and continue for more than 30 years, as well as women who get migraines with aura, are less likely to have a type of breast cancer that is positive for a trait called estrogen receptor (ER+). One theory proposes that the hormone estrogen plays a role because estrogen is known to be a migraine trigger. Another is that women who get migraines tend to avoid things such as alcohol, which is known to increase breast cancer risk. Doctors admit that the relationship is complicated, and they are cautious about making conclusions about this link.

to enter this field of research. Neurologist Joel Saper expressed optimism about the new initiative:

> *While research in adult migraine is grossly under-funded, the study of migraine in children has been almost completely neglected. In fact, many people are completely unaware that children suffer from migraine. Also, pharmacological treatment geared toward this younger population is rarely investigated, and physicians struggle with adapting adult treatments to kids.*[33]

Experts hope that as more research is done on migraines, they will be able to provide better information and care to people of all ages.

Chapter One:
Understanding Migraines

1. Mayo Clinic Staff, "Tension Headache," Mayo Clinic, August 19, 2017. www.mayoclinic. org/diseases-conditions/tension-headache/ symptoms-causes/syc-20353977.

2. Mayo Clinic Staff, "Migraine," Mayo Clinic, April 26, 2017. www.mayoclinic.org/ diseases-conditions/migraine-headache/ symptoms-causes/syc-20360201.

3. Deborah Weaver, interview by Anne K. Brown, July 2, 2009.

4. Tammy Rome, "Migraine Gets on My Nerves," Migraine.com, October 5, 2016. migraine.com/ living-migraine/gets-on-my-nerves/.

Chapter Two:
Differences Among Migraines

5. Quoted in "Breakthrough in Migraine Genetics," Medical News Today, April 18, 2008. www.medicalnewstoday.com/articles/ 104589.php.

6. Jerry W. Swanson, MD, "Ocular Migraine: When to Seek Help," Mayo Clinic, August 10, 2017. www.mayoclinic.org/diseases-conditions/migraine-headache/expert-answers/ocular-migraine/faq-20058113.

7. Swanson, "Ocular Migraine."

8. Paula Dumas, "7 Types of Migraine: Which Do You Have?," Migraine Again, March 9, 2015.

migraineagain.com/10-types-of-migraine
-which-do-you-have/.

9. Jennifer Robinson, MD, "What Are Vestibular Migraines?," WebMD, February 24, 2016. www.webmd.com/migraines-headaches/vestibular-migraines#1.

10. Anna Eidt, "Why the 'Migraine Personality' Is Total Bunk," Migraine.com, September 16, 2016. migraine.com/living-migraine/why-the-migraine-personality-is-total-bunk/.

11. Eidt, "Why the 'Migraine Personality' Is Total Bunk."

12. Quoted in Michael John Coleman and Terri Miller Burchfield, "Migraines: Myth vs. Reality," M.A.G.N.U.M., accessed November 22, 2017. www.migraines.org/myth/mythreal.htm.

13. Marilyn Hartman, interview by Anne K. Brown, July 19, 2009.

14. Nancy Mildebrandt, interview by Anne K. Brown, July 18, 2009.

Chapter Three: Managing Migraines

15. Wayne Hoffmann, interview by Anne K. Brown, August 20, 2009.

16. Quoted in Pauline Anderson, "Identifying Migraine 'Protectors,'" Medscape, June 23, 2016. www.medscape.com/viewarticle/865283.

17. Quoted in "NFL Films Presents Top Ten Gutsiest Performances: Terrell Davis," NFL. www.nfl.com/videos/nfl-films-presents/09000d5d810a5972/Top-Ten-Gutsiest- Performances-Terrell-Davis.

Chapter Four:
Treating Migraines

18. Laurie Tarkan, "5 Natural Headache Remedies," *Prevention*, April 25, 2012. www.prevention.com/health/health-concerns/natural-cures-pain-5-natural-headache-remedies.

19. Miya Kressin, interview by Anne K. Brown, July 14, 2009.

20. Hansa Bhargava, "Does Acupuncture Work? A Quick Review of the Latest Evidence," Medscape, July 5, 2017. www.medscape.com/viewarticle/882127.

21. Michael Shames, "SCAM ALERT: *'The Migraine Protocol'* Could Give You Headaches," San Diego Consumers' Action Network, January 26, 2015. www.sandiegocan.org/2015/01/26/scam-alert-migraine-protocol-causes-headaches-than-it-relieves/.

22. Shames, "SCAM ALERT."

23. Shames, "SCAM ALERT."

24. Deborah Weaver, interview by Anne K. Brown, July 2, 2009.

25. "Facts About Triptans," National Headache Foundation, November 19, 2007. www.headaches.org/2007/11/19/facts-about-triptans/#How_Triptans_Work.

Chapter Five:
Continuing Research

26. Joel Saper, "Migraine Research Foundation Launches with Announcement of First Annual Research Grants." stanford.wellsphere.com/

migraine-headaches-article/great-news-from-the-migraine-research-foundation/212789.

27. Neil Lava, MD, "Would TMS Help Your Migraine?," WebMD, May 30, 2017. www.webmd.com/migraines-headaches/tms-for-migraines#1.

28. Lava, "Would TMS Help Your Migraines?"

29. "Is Plastic Surgery the Hail Mary Play for Battling Migraines?," Healthline, accessed November 30, 2017. www.healthline.com/health/plastic-surgery-botox-migraines#1.

30. James Gallagher, "Migraine Therapy That Cut Attacks Hailed as 'Huge Deal,'" BBC News, November 30, 2017. www.bbc.com/news/health-42154668.

31. Gallagher, "Migraine Therapy That Cut Attacks Hailed as 'Huge Deal.'"

32. Anna Reynolds, "Smoking Marijuana Is the Only Thing That Makes My Migraines Go Away," *Self*, July 2, 2016. www.self.com/story/smoking-marijuana-is-the-only-thing-that-makes-my-migraines-go-away.

33. Quoted in "Pediatric Migraine: New Initiative to Support Research," Medical News Today, March 23, 2009. www.medicalnewstoday.com/articles/143222.php.

aneurysm: An abnormal swelling or ballooning of an artery wall.

aura: A disturbance in vision commonly experienced by migraine patients. It may include bright flashes, sparkling lines or zigzags, or blind spots.

clinical trial: A testing procedure to study the effectiveness and side effects of a new drug or medical treatment.

constriction: The narrowing or compression of a blood vessel.

dehydration: The loss of water from the body due to sweating or lack of fluid consumption.

diagnosis: A doctor's assessment and identification of a patient's illness or injury.

dilation: The widening of a blood vessel.

inflammation: An increase in blood flow to tissues, which causes swelling and pain.

menopause: The process women experience when their menstrual cycle permanently ceases.

nausea: Stomach upset that leads to the feeling that vomiting is likely.

over-the-counter (OTC) medicine: A medication that can be purchased without a doctor's prescription.

puberty: The time period in which children mature physically and girls first begin menstruation.

stroke: A blockage within a blood vessel that deprives part of the brain of oxygen, which may cause disability or death.

symptom: A physical change in the body that is associated with an illness.

American Migraine Foundation
19 Mantua Road
Mt. Royal, NJ 08061
(856) 423-0043
amf@talley.com
americanmigrainefoundation.org
This organization's website offers educational
information for headache sufferers, including migraine
management, treatment options, and recent research.

Migraine Adventure
2 Emerson Road
Kintraw, PA31 6JR
United Kingdom
www.migraineadventure.org.uk
This British organization provides information on how
to avoid migraines, tips young adults can use to tell their
friends about their migraines, and general information.

**Migraine Awareness Group: A National
Understanding for Migraineurs (MAGNUM)**
100 N. Union Street, Suite B
Alexandria, VA 22314
(703) 349-1929
www.migraines.org
Also known as the National Migraine Association,
MAGNUM offers information and links about all
aspects of migraines. An online community is available
to allow chatting among migraine sufferers. Always ask
a parent or guardian before participating in any kind of
online forum.

National Headache Foundation
820 N. Orleans Street, Suite 201
Chicago, IL 60610
(312) 274-2650
info@headaches.org
www.headaches.org
The foundation's website offers information to help manage migraines, tips for talking to a health care provider, and updates on clinical trials.

FOR MORE INFORMATION

Books

Buchholz, David. *Heal Your Headache*. New York, NY: Workman, 2002.
This book provides a doctor's tips for dealing with headaches through diet, exercise, and lifestyle. Since everyone's body and migraines are different, these tips may work for some people but not for others. Any changes should first be discussed with a doctor to make sure they will not be harmful to other aspects of a person's health.

Ford-Martin, Paula. *The Everything Health Guide to Migraines*. Avon, MA: Adams Media, 2008.
This guidebook helps readers understand and deal with migraines; it is written in language for ordinary people, not just doctors.

Moe, Barbara. *Everything You Need to Know About Migraines and Other Headaches*. New York, NY: Rosen, 2000.
This is an easy-to-read reference about understanding the diagnosis and treatment of migraines.

Robert, Teri. *Living Well with Migraine Disease and Headache*. New York, NY: HarperCollins, 2005.
The author provides tips to make life easier for those suffering from migraines.

Votava, Andrea. *Coping with Migraines and Other Headaches*. New York, NY: Rosen, 2000.
This common-sense guide for teens helps them understand and cope with their own headaches as well as those of family members.

Websites

KidsHealth
kidshealth.org
This website has different areas for parents, kids, and teens and explains how the human body works as well as how to stay healthy.

Mayo Clinic
www.mayoclinic.org
The highly respected Mayo Clinic maintains this website, which explains various medical matters—including migraines—in everyday language and includes a question-and-answer section.

MigrainePal: "Migraine With Aura Symptoms, Triggers & Treatment"
www.blog.migrainepal.com/blog/2015/8/6/migraine-with-aura-symptoms-triggers-treatment
This website provides information about auras, including pictures of what many people see when they experience an aura.

Migraine Research Foundation: Find a Doctor
migraineresearchfoundation.org/resources/find-a-doctor/
The Migraine Research Foundation keeps an updated list of headache specialists in the United States for adults as well as for kids and teens.

Why Does My Head Hurt?
www.webmd.com/migraines-headaches/headache-map-tool/default.htm
This WebMD headache map tool allows users to designate where their head hurts most and how often the headaches occur. It gives possible causes for the headaches and advice on whether or not the person should see a doctor. This tool is not intended to diagnose headache disorders, only to help give people more information about them.

A

acetaminophen (Tylenol), 6, 23, 70–72, 74
acupuncture, 67–68
alcohol, 11, 14, 26, 41, 44, 89
allodynia, 48
alternative treatments, 65–68
antibody therapy, 86–87
antidepressants, 76–77
antiseizure medications, 77
anxiety, 12, 17, 35, 50, 51, 52, 56, 65
aromatherapy, 78
aspirin, 10, 23, 70–72, 74
auras, 14, 15–17, 30–32, 34, 74, 89

B

beta blockers, 75
biofeedback, **77–78**
Botox, 75–76, 84
brain, examining the, 18–20, 81
brain stem, 18–19, 21
brain tumor, 11, 12
breast cancer, 89

C

caffeine, 11, 42, 74
calcium channel blocker, 75
cerebellum, 18, 19
cerebrum, 18–19, 22
children, migraines and, 28, 31–32, 38, 55–56, 88–89
cluster headaches, 12, 13–14, 76
common migraine, 30
complex migraines, 16, 30, 74
cortical spreading depression (CSD), 21

D

daith piercing, 78–79
Davis, Terrell, 7, 48–49, 72
depression, 15, 46, 52, 65, 76–77
DHE (dihydroergotamine), 86
diet, 62–64
dizziness, 17, 30–33, 46, 72, 74–75
doctor
    common questions asked by, 10
    when to see a, 23

drugs
  addiction to, 56, 73, 74
  illegal, 11, 87

E

emotional effects of migraines, 51–52, 70
emotional support, 70
exercise, 64

F

familial hemiplegic migraine (FHM), 29–30
folk remedies, 58–59
foods as triggers, 41–42, 45
frovatriptan (Frova), 73

G

genes/genetic link for migraines, 28–30
guilt, 50–52, 70

H

headaches
  primary headaches, 8–9, 11–14
  secondary headaches, 8–12
  as symptoms, 9–11
head injuries, 39–40
hormones, 26, 32, 40, 45, 52, 89

I

ibuprofen (Advil), 6, 23, 70–72
International Classification of Headache Disorders (ICHD),
  30, 32

J

journal, keeping a, 45–47, 57, 64

L

lifestyle changes, 61–64
light, sensitivity to (photophobia), 13–14, 17–18, 27, 37–38, 73

M

marijuana, medical, 87–88
massage, 67
medications, 60–62, 70–77, 86
  abortive treatments, 60
  cost of, 52–55
  generic vs. name brand, 53
  off-label, 75–77
  over-the-counter (OTC), 6, 23, 39, 42, 61, 70–72, 74
  rebound headaches and, 56
  triptans, 73–74
meditation, 65–66

men, migraines and, 26, 33, 64
meninges, 18, 20, 22
menstrual cycle, 26, 32, 40
mental disorders/illness, 4, 51–52
migraine equivalent, 31
"migraine personality," 33–34
Migraine Research Foundation, 80, 88
migraines
    biological sex and, 26, 33
    classification, 30–33
    diagnosing, 23–25, 74
    effect on everyday life, 49–51
    family history of, 24, 28–29
    general information about, 6, 8, 14, 17
    managing/preventing, 7, 36, 38–39, 43–57, 60, 62
    misinformation about, 7–8, 28, 33–35, 51, 80
    new research and technology, 7, 80–89
    patterns, 6, 45–46
    recognition of as medical condition, 6–8
    stages, 14–18
    study of, 7, 18, 21–22
    symptoms/characteristics, 15–16, 17–18, 26–27, 46
    theories about, 20–23
    treatment, 6, 17, 21, 44–45, 49, 52, 57–79
    triggers, 35–43, 44–46, 48, 60, 65, 89
migraine with brain stem aura, 31–32
motion sickness, 36, 40

N
nausea, 6, 17, 27, 33–34, 56, 72, 74
new daily persistent headaches (NDPH), 12, 14
NSAIDs, 72

O
occipital nerve stimulation, 82
ocular migraine, 30
opioid problem, 73

P
physical therapy, 67
picture, drawing to describe migraine, 47–48
plastic surgery, 84–85
postdrome, 18
primary headaches, 8–9, 11–12
    types of, 12–14
prodrome, 15

R
rebound headaches, 56, 62

retinal migraine, 30

S

scams, avoiding, 68–70
secondary headaches, 8–12, 24, 27
seizure, 32, 81
serotonin, 20, 22–23, 52, 75
sleep, migraines and, 15, 37, 39, 45, 64
smells, as migraine trigger, 39, 45
smoking, 45
sound, sensitivity to (phonophobia), 13–14, 17–18, 27, 37–38,
    45, 73
SPECT scan, 81
stress, 12–15, 33, 34, 36, 47, 50, 65
    types of, 36–37
stroke, 12, 16–17, 31, 70, 81
sumatriptan (Imitrex), 53, 73
symptom, defined, 9

T

tai chi, 66–67
tension headaches, 12–14
thalamus, 18, 20
tracking migraines, 44–47
transcranial magnetic stimulation (TMS), 21, 82–84
transient ischemic attach (TIA), 16–17
trigeminal nerve, 21–22
triggers, migraine, 26, 35–45, 48, 60, 65, 89
triptans, 73–74

U

unproven treatments, 77–79

V

vision changes/disturbances, 6, 12, 14–17, 30–31
vomiting, 13, 17, 27, 32

W

weather, effect on migraines, 26, 32, 36, 39, 45, 46
women, migraines and, 23, 26, 33, 40, 89

Y

yoga, 66–67

Z

zolmitriptan (Zomig), 54, 55, 73

Jennifer Lombardo earned her BA in English from the University at Buffalo and still resides in Buffalo, New York, with her cat, Chip. She has helped write a number of books for young adults on topics ranging from world history to body image. In her spare time, she enjoys cross-stitching, hiking, and volunteering with local organizations.